Dana E. King, MD
Melissa H. Hunter, MD
Jerri R. Harris, MPH

Dealing with the Psychological and Spiritual Aspects of Menopause
Finding Hope in the Midlife

Pre-publication
REVIEWS,
COMMENTARIES,
EVALUATIONS . . .

"This book fills a missing niche in the menopause literature through its emphasis on the spiritual link of this life-changing transition in women's lives. When we look in our hearts and in the medical literature, we know that life passages, health events, and discomfort are all moments for seeking a larger vision of life—menopause is a combination of all three of those moments. The authors force us to examine this perspective and, in so doing, 'de'-medicalize menopause. I remember a patient telling me about his wife going through 'the great interchange of life,' and this book made me reflect on how the greatest interchange we can hope for is a connection to the spiritual. In that context, we, as women and health care providers, must provide 'soul care'—assistance and permission to women to allow them to care for themselves and their souls during this time. The authors provide many practical suggestions for such care as well as strong evidence for the influence of our American culture on 'symptoms.' This simply and clearly written book, with its combination of fact and hope, provides a wonderful opportunity for practitioners and patients to reconsider menopause and, in so doing, change the image of women's aging from remorse for the past to one of hope for the future."

Peggy J. Wagner, PhD
*Associate Professor
and Director of Research,
Department of Family Medicine,
Medical College of Georgia*

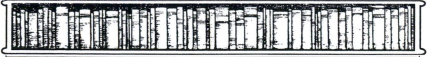

"**A** practical, easy-to-read book that provides a refreshing look at menopause and midlife. The authors emphasize that menopause is, as with other life phases, a natural transition and embodies the whole of life experiences— an important concept for women, and those who care about them, to remember. The book separates fact from myth, makes recommendations, provides additional resources to access, and overall will enhance a woman's capacity to deal with this midlife transition that all women experience. Most important, the book takes a whole-person approach, dealing with the biopsychosocial and spiritual aspects of a woman's life. The end analysis of the authors and hopefully of those who read this book is that women who go through menopause are capable of positive growth and a new perspective on life. This book is designed to bring hope to women—'a hope that can sustain you through the challenges of midlife and beyond.'"

Ann C. Jobe, MD, MSN
Dean and Professor of Family Medicine,
Mercer University School of Medicine

The Haworth Pastoral Press®
An Imprint of The Haworth Press, Inc.
New York • London • Oxford

Dealing with the Psychological and Spiritual Aspects of Menopause
Finding Hope in the Midlife

THE HAWORTH PASTORAL PRESS®
Religion and Mental Health
Harold G. Koenig, MD
Senior Editor

Dealing with the Psychological and Spiritual Aspects of Menopause
Finding Hope in the Midlife

Dana E. King, MD
Melissa H. Hunter, MD
Jerri R. Harris, MPH

The Haworth Pastoral Press®
An Imprint of The Haworth Press, Inc.
New York • London • Oxford

For more information on this book or to order, visit
http://www.haworthpress.com/store/product.asp?sku=5378

or call 1-800-HAWORTH (800-429-6784) in the United States and Canada
or (607) 722-5857 outside the United States and Canada

or contact orders@HaworthPress.com

The Haworth Pastoral Press®, an imprint of The Haworth Press, Inc., 10 Alice Street, Binghamton, NY 13904-1580.

Cover design by Lora Wiggins.

Library of Congress Cataloging-in-Publication Data

King, Dana E.
    Dealing with the psychological and spiritual aspects of menopause : finding hope in the midlife / Dana E. King, Melissa H. Hunter, Jerri R. Harris.
        p. cm.
    Includes bibliographical references and index.
    ISBN 0-7890-2303-2 (hard : alk. paper) — ISBN 0-7890-2304-0 (soft : alk. paper)
    1. Menopause—Psychological aspects. I. Hunter, Melissa. II. Harris, Jerri R. III. Title.

RG186.K535 2005
618.1'75'0019—dc22

2004020327

To Jane, who remained spiritually strong
in the face of adversity

ABOUT THE AUTHORS

Dana E. King, MD, is a family physician and researcher with a career-long interest in spirituality and women's health. He received his medical degree at the University of Kentucky and completed specialty residency training in Family Medicine at the University of Maryland in Baltimore. He also completed an academic fellowship at the University of North Carolina at Chapel Hill. Dr. King is currently Associate Professor of Family Medicine at the Medical University of South Carolina. He has been widely published in the areas of spirituality, women's health issues, and obstetrics. His first book, *Faith, Spirituality, and Medicine* (Haworth), was highly acclaimed as a concise and useful text and one of the first textbooks for health professionals in the emerging field of spirituality and medicine.

Melissa H. Hunter, MD, is Associate Professor in the Department of Family Medicine, Medical University of South Carolina College of Medicine, Charleston. She received her medical degree from the Medical University of South Carolina College of Medicine, and completed a residency in family medicine at McLeod Regional Medical Center in Florence, South Carolina. Dr. Hunter also completed a faculty development fellowship at the University of North Carolina at Chapel Hill School of Medicine.

Jerri R. Harris, MPH, is a medical writer, editor, and educator, recently retired from the Brody School of Medicine (Department of Family Medicine) at East Carolina University in Greenville, North Carolina. She writes on numerous health topics, including prenatal care, adolescent health, and women's health. Ms. Harris has taught scientific writing and has presented seminars on male-female communication issues and writing medical information for patients. She has received recognition from the American Academy of Neurology for production of the CD-ROM *Family Practice Curriculum in Neurology.*

CONTENTS

Foreword

Compared to other books on the topic of menopause, this book is a welcome surprise. It goes beyond the usual "herbs and hormones" approach to treating menopausal symptoms and addresses ways in which women may come to peace with changes they face at midlife. Even more remarkable is the way the authors emphasize that menopause can be, and frequently is, a positive experience for women.

From the perspectives of my practice as a family physician, my self as a midlife woman, and my journey as a woman of faith, this book addresses many questions that other works have omitted. We are often afraid to discuss spiritual matters in the medical setting, yet it is the soul and spirit that govern the way we feel every day. Every person believes in something, whether as complex as a formalized religion or as simple as the basic goodness (or not) of humankind. These beliefs have a profound influence over every aspect of our lives—including our physical health. The authors remind us that expectations about menopause profoundly affect women's experiences with menopause.

As a child I remember hearing my aunts calling it "minipause"—but they did not say much more. In the South of 1960s' America, bodily functions were spoken of euphemistically if at all, and never in polite company. We now monitor television carefully to avoid having to explain erectile dysfunction to preteens, yet menopause is still a taboo subject in many places. When a woman comes to me and confesses, "I know you are going to think I am crazy, but . . .," I am glad to let her know that there are safe places to talk, ask, and, yes, safe places to cry. Tears are good for the soul, and a sympathetic ear offered by someone with knowledge about menopause can guide a woman toward positive feelings and actions.

The advice about nutrition and exercise in this book is clear and useful. Physical activity and a prudent diet are the foundations of health at any age, and the authors provide an excellent overview of the knowledge and strategies for achieving both. Even the most overscheduled person can find in this book the inspiration to set aside 30 of the 1,440 minutes in each day to take care of ourselves and to make food choices that will strengthen bones and build muscles instead of "saddlebags."

In our younger years, many of us were so focused on *doing* that we did not think much about *being*. We defined our selves by what we did, how we looked, and by other external measures. As menstrual periods stop and body parts begin to sag, we are forced to redefine our physical selves in our own minds. It is important to look at our existential selves at this time as well. Pondering the questions "What does this mean to me?" and "What are my choices now?" can lead to new perspectives on life and our place in it. This book provides useful tools for addressing these questions.

Many women in today's society have few opportunities to discuss their feelings about menopause with other women. Demands of full-time employment outside the home coupled with household responsibilities have left many of my patients (and their doctors) with minimal free time to engage in these conversations. I suspect that many of the concerns women bring to their physicians or therapists are those that were once shared and resolved at the kitchen table with sisters or friends.

We often also find ourselves too busy to grieve the losses, both great and small, that populate our lives. Grief unacknowledged, and thus unresolved, is associated with much of the depression experienced by the women I treat in my medical practice. Some are dragged down by past events that they have been unable to release, some are holding grudges against another, and many are carrying personal (false) guilt over uncontrollable events. Forgiveness is the foundation of a peaceful existence, yet we often find the greatest difficulty in forgiving ourselves.

Although faith can allow us to find forgiveness, religion can sometimes be toxic. So much mythology has grown around the central truths of many religions that the themes of love, joy, and grace have been hidden. For example, some religious groups assign very specific social rules and gender roles to followers, and those who live their lives otherwise may feel guilty because they perceive themselves as falling short of expectations. Women may be chastised for seeking treatment for depression, having been told that a faith that is strong enough will prevent depression, worry, sickness, divorce, misbehaving children, and other conditions that are common in human existence. Guilt added to grief can be the final straw, but healthy faith and practice can provide the keys to new meanings, a greater sense of self-honor and respect, and the best health of a woman's life.

Why counseling? Changes in thinking patterns can profoundly alter a woman's concept of herself. After feeling bad for a long time she may believe that she can never feel better. If she struggles with tasks she may believe she is no longer competent. A good therapist can help her unlearn self-defeating thought patterns that are a product of her symptoms and guide her in the process of self-discovery at this transitional time of her life. The authors explain the various counseling options available to women in a way that clarifies the major differences in the therapists a woman might choose.

As I often share with my menopausal patients, "This won't kill you, but it can drive you nuts!" Hope lies in finding meaning in life events: "What can I learn from this, and what can it show me about myself and the world?" There is wisdom to be gleaned from any situation, no matter how negative it may seem at the time. The authors of this book provide welcome ways to cope, survive, and, yes, even thrive during this transition.

May your reading of it be blessed.

Janice Daugherty, MD
Associate Professor, Department of Family Medicine
Brody School of Medicine, East Carolina University
Greenville, North Carolina

Preface

So why write a book about menopause? Try this experiment. Go to your local bookstore and look at the books in the women's health section. You will see that more than half of the books deal with menopause, focusing on estrogen, hormones, and osteoporosis. You will also find a few books about vitamins, supplements, and alternative therapies but fewer still on the main problem that women face during the midlife—stress.

The following scenario illustrates how the stress women face in the midlife years is often discovered. My (DK) wife will ask me when I come home, "How many women did you make cry today?" It is not that I *made* them cry, it is just that they could not hold in the stress and emotion any longer. The women were able to hold themselves together at home, on the way to the doctor's office, at the registration desk, and even while the nurse took their blood pressure. Then I come through the door. "Hi, I'm Dr. King. What brings you here today?" The dam bursts and the tears come rolling down their cheeks, then the sobs.

"What's going on?" I ask.

"Nothing."

Then the big sigh.

They begin to tell me their stories: the kids having trouble in school, the nonsupportive alcoholic husband, the sick mother with the stroke who just moved in with them, their inability to deal with situations as well as they used to, and sometimes I almost cry too.

That is why we wrote this book. We wanted to help women during this particularly stressful time. We wanted to share our experience in working with women in midlife who are dealing with anxiety, stress, and depression, as well as to elaborate on other psychological and spiritual aspects of menopause. There is much to share—more than we can squeeze into a twenty-minute office visit. We want to let you know there is hope. The scientific break-throughs of the past few years have provided better insight into the problems women face. New medications are available to treat anxiety and depression, and recent research on the link between spiritual and emotional health confirms our belief in the great need to deal with the spiritual aspects of the midlife as well.

We will not spend much time discussing estrogen and other hormone therapies. This is not because they are not relevant, but because other books are available that address these issues. The most important way to discuss the topic of hormones is with your doctor, weighing your individual risks and benefits carefully.

We want to focus more on what we see most in the office—the emotional toll of menopause and the midlife. We want to focus on hope, on where one can go for help with stress and worry, on which medicines and counseling techniques work best, and on addressing the spiritual issues that have been neglected in the past. So sit back, give the kids some money to go to the movies, tell your husband he *can* go play golf today, and read this book. You will know more, feel better, and be more prepared to face tomorrow.

We sincerely hope that the discussion in the chapters that follow will provide new avenues for finding peace and hope to sustain you through the challenges of midlife and beyond.

Acknowledgments

I want to thank Kathy, Karen, and Steven for their constant love and support. I thank Lisa and Jerri for their help and dedication.

—DK

Thanks a million to Chuck, Gareth, and Hannah Claire for all their continued love and support.

—MH

To my husband, Brian, and my daughter, Kendra, who were constant and loving companions on my menopause journey. Thank you.

—JH

Introduction

Many issues can collide to cause enormous stress on the midlife woman during menopause, such as physical changes, emotional stress, medical illness, and psychological health. Menopause is a psychological and spiritual life event. Apprehension, mood swings, feelings of grief, and family change often accompany the midlife, and can be more intensified when a woman also faces her own serious illness. Anxiety may come from many places, including physical changes, sexual changes, children leaving home, emotional ups and downs, and uncertainty about how to deal with difficult medical decisions.

Most women experiencing menopause do not become seriously physically ill as a result, but different factors do combine during midlife to produce a greater risk of depression, emotional instability, and self-doubt. The effects of aging, the empty nest syndrome, and social changes compound the physiological effects of menopause. You were once busy taking kids to and from various activities. Now you are faced with teenagers who can drive themselves everywhere, and at all hours. As the teens face tremendous challenges and temptations from smoking, drugs, and sexual pressures and need your advice, your mother becomes sick and requires attention. Then you turn to your husband (if you have one) only to discover he is having a midlife crisis of his own—doubting his career and self-worth just when you need someone to be strong to bolster you. Whether many of the psychological stresses are caused by hormonal changes is the subject of many books and much research, but this may not be the most important issue for many women. The most important issue is how to face the multitude of spiritual and psychological challenges that pile up during the perimenopausal years.

This book addresses the many challenges women face in midlife, with special attention to the spiritual and psychological needs during this life stage. It focuses on the early midlife years of menopause because of the unique confluence of factors that women face during this time. The authors draw from their spiritual and medical backgrounds to find hope for women who face these challenges. Women from different backgrounds or spiritual traditions will be able to derive hope from the inspiring stories from patients and from learning more about the mind/body/spirit connection that is so important to health at midlife.

The first chapter, "The Transition to Menopause: The Journey Begins," is an overview from both the medical and the social points of view of the challenges of menopause as a time of transition. Menopause is a developmental stage in the life cycle during which women gradually adapt to biological, social, psychological, and spiritual changes that come with decreasing ovarian function. This can be a time of great uncertainty. When a woman misses only one or two periods she cannot be certain that her cycles have completely stopped. Menstrual cycles may be irregular for a year or more in the perimenopausal period. Along with the well-recognized biological transition from high estrogen levels and menstrual periods to low estrogen and no menstruation, significant psychological transitions occur during midlife as well. A woman may be dealing with changing relationships with children, marital problems or widowhood, or the illness or loss of parents. On the positive side, menopause can also be a time of transition from childbearing and child rearing to a time of personal growth and many newfound freedoms.

Chapter 2, "Closing and Opening Doors: Dealing with a Journey of Personal Loss," is not only for those who have recently lost a loved one. Feelings about children leaving home, divorce, or loss of function in parents may be similar to the emotional and psychological effects of the death of a close relative. These emotional burdens on top of the physical and physiological changes during menopause can sometimes seem too much to bear. Talking to partners, friends, and relatives about the unique emotional stress that occurs during midlife may help increase insight into the extra need for emotional support. For many women, the spiritual perspective that faith brings can sometimes be the only place where grief can find peace.

Chapter 3, "Mood and the Mind in Menopause," discusses the stress and strain on moods and attitudes as well as the greater risk of depression in women during midlife. It also provides some information about recent breakthroughs in treatment. The chapter includes a review of sexuality at menopause, including a discussion of why most women find sex more satisfying in the menopausal years.

Women suffer a greater burden of mood disorders than do men. Throughout her lifetime a woman is twice as likely as a man to have depression. Happily married women experience less major depression than single women, but other factors can contribute to depression. These include sexual abuse, a history of domestic violence, miscarriage or abortion, death of a child or spouse, family history of depression, or even being the mother of a child with attention deficit disorder. Cultural influences may also affect the risk of depression. Women face many, and often conflicting, roles as mother, spouse, and breadwinner. Such concerns as sexual harassment in the workplace or unequal pay with lack of advancement compared to male co-workers place women at a greater risk of depression. As this chapter will show, finding help from psychological and spiritual sources can be a vital addition to medical treatment.

Both counseling and medication may help during the transition to menopause. Hormone replacement may relieve some of the physiological symptoms, but it may not help with other stresses and symptoms. The most effective ways to treat the psychological symptoms of menopause are medication, exercise, and counseling.

Depression may be treated with antidepressants, such as selective serotonin reuptake inhibitors (SSRIs), even as potential hormone imbalances are still being tested. Counseling combined with medication is best for many women, particularly if a woman is so depressed that she becomes suicidal, or is experiencing marriage or family conflicts, or is so disabled that she cannot work if she is employed. Women who have strong religious beliefs should seek treatment from someone who will include spiritual counseling in treatment. Research has shown that people with strong religious beliefs respond better when spiritual aspects are included with therapy. Women may need to overcome the opinion held by some in society and religions that depression is a sign of a weak personality or weak faith. Religious and spiritual women can consider modern medicines as an answer to prayer, not as something to avoid.

As with depression, anxiety disorders are more common for women than for men. They may include generalized anxiety disorder, panic disorder, and phobias. A variety of medications are available to treat anxiety disorders.

Counseling plays a key role for women facing the challenges of menopause and is helpful in many situations. Chapter 4, "Counseling and Group Support," presents the benefits of counseling for women with stress or conflict in their marriage, in their homes, or in their workplaces. Counseling also can help with specific anxiety disorders and depression, either alone or with medication. Referral to a psychiatrist or family therapist may be an option for women who have severe depression, psychosis, or intense marital conflict. Spiritual issues and conflicts, self-doubt, and feeling abandoned by one's religion or faith can be seriously harmful to overall health but are often the last issues discussed in a clinical setting. Individual or group counseling, support groups with other women, and focused self-care without guilt can help restore balance during midlife.

Exercise is another important therapy that has not received enough emphasis. Chapter 5, "Exercise: Moving Along the Menopause Journey," recommends regular exercise for menopausal and midlife women. Walking, running, or jogging can increase bone density without increasing the risk of osteoarthritis. Exercise can also help treat anxiety and depression. Walking every day and changing routines, such as parking farther from workplaces and stores (called *lifestyle walking*), are as effective as more structured programs. In fact, walking at a moderate pace for as little as two to three hours a week will benefit health and may even reduce the chance of becoming depressed.

Chapter 6, "Menopause and the Workplace," discusses managing menopause in the workplace, perhaps one of the most challenging midlife experiences for women. Although expressed less openly now than in the past, women's value at work, as in our culture, has often been judged on youth and sexual attractiveness. Women are often thought of as having less value as they age. As a result, many women find the menopausal experience at work to be stressful, and they look for ways to manage symptoms without drawing attention to themselves.

Although menopause still can increase stress and anxiety at work, attitudes toward women gradually have become more open and accepting in recent years. Some major companies are now including menopause as a topic of health and wellness seminars in the workplace. More attention to women's health and menopause in the media has helped both men and women gain more accurate information about menopause and the related health risks of midlife. More choices for women, more recognition of the stresses women face, and more research on the psychological and spiritual aspects of health have helped to provide renewed hope for women in the midlife, even in the workplace.

Chapter 7, "Spiritual Issues Facing Women at Midlife," focuses more fully on spiritual aspects of midlife, including spiritual issues and special challenges during the perimenopausal period. What do we mean by *spiritual?* Spiritual aspects of menopause deal with a woman's view of herself in the context of a broader perspective of her world and her faith. *Religion* or *religious* refers to a more formal set of beliefs and practices shared with others. Women's religious and spiritual beliefs play an important role in their views of life and often become even more important when they also face serious medical illness. Under stress, some may forget the important role that their spiritual and religious views play in providing a context for thinking about the meaning of life changes or illness. Not considering one's spiritual and religious beliefs when facing the emotional and psychological stresses that come during midlife can frustrate the process of dealing with these stresses. Discussing spiritual coping with health care providers about menopausal issues may help identify an important source of strength.

Menopause and the early midlife period are often psychological and spiritual life events as well as physical and physiological events. Depression, anxiety, mood swings, feelings of grief, and family change are common. Most women who go through menopause are not seriously physically ill as a result, but cultural expectations about aging and appearance often have a profound effect on women's self-esteem during this period.

In the chapters that follow we explore the psychological and spiritual aspects of the midlife as a means of countering the despair and fatigue that often come with menopause. In their place, we seek to promote personal growth and a new outlook for many women, one that is filled with hope.

Chapter 1

The Transition to Menopause: The Journey Begins

A woman's experience during the transition to menopause depends on many factors, including general physical and emotional health, diet, levels of physical activity, and social support. Some women may view the transition as the beginning of old age and loss of status in a society that values youth, beauty, and vitality. At first a woman may react to this "change of life" with anger or sadness, focusing on lost opportunities or a life in decline. As time passes women are more likely to feel hope and possibility, viewing this stage of life as an opportunity for growth and a renewed sense of self.

Balancing these physical uncertainties and the emotional and psychological experiences can be a challenge during menopause because so much seems to be happening at the same time. Understanding how the body functions can help ease much of the uncertainty about the physical changes. A number of options are available to relieve symptoms, beginning with a discussion with a health care provider about medications that may help. The emotional and psychological experiences likely will require additional attention.

Sharing experiences with other women can be of great importance in gaining perspective, particularly when sharing with others is combined with reflection on one's own possibilities in moving toward the next third of life. Perhaps the greatest long-term benefit will come from tending to religious or spiritual needs to achieve balance amid all of the physical and emotional changes at peri-menopause. For some women this may mean reaffirming relation-ships at church and making more time to spend with friends. The mind/body/spirit connection is powerful and healing. Combining regular exercise or yoga with prayer or meditation also helps in-crease feelings of well-being and peace. Other measures that can help are deep-breathing exercises, taking a leisurely bath or hav-ing a massage, or walking alone or with a friend in a park or other natural setting. These simple activities help quiet the mind and in-vite a healthier perspective on all the changes taking place, de-crease feelings of anxiety, and help restore spiritual balance.

IS MENOPAUSE A DISEASE?

Throughout her lifetime after puberty a woman is more likely than a man to seek medical care, often related to reproductive is-sues. In part because she uses health care more often, a woman's health issues are more likely to be medicalized than a man's. Ad-vances in medical treatment have provided great relief, but in the process doctors and their patients have come to expect that many life events are medical conditions that must be treated and cured.

Menopause is not a disease; it is a natural process every woman will experience if she lives into her fifties. Knowing the difference between menopausal symptoms and feelings that are influenced by other health or life circumstances can help maintain perspec-tive on the process. The transition to menopause certainly has a way of getting a woman's attention. Beyond the physical changes, many women find that it can also be a time of reflection, reassess-ment, and renewal of purpose. More than a transition, menopause can hold the surprising power of transformation and can lead to a more meaningful life. We have included more on how that can happen in later chapters. But first, the following is a brief review of the menopausal process and how other women have dealt with it.

WHEN DOES MENOPAUSE BEGIN?

Menopause begins at different times for different women. It has several stages: premenopause, which includes all reproductive years leading to the transition; perimenopause, when symptoms begin; menopause, medically one year after the final menstrual period; and postmenopause, the years of a woman's life after menopause. The phrase "going through" menopause can be misleading because the process is not a predictable phasing in and out of each stage. Some of the symptoms may occur for at least a year after menopause. Perimenopause can last from 1 to 10 years, the average being 4.8 years. The average age of perimenopause is 47.5, although the range can be from the late thirties to the mid-fifties. A number of factors influence when perimenopause begins and how long it lasts. For example, women who smoke tend to enter perimenopause up to two years earlier and have a shorter perimenopause than nonsmokers.

Women enter the menopausal years with assumptions that have been shaped by society and their own expectations. How a woman views menopause depends in large part on understanding the process as much as on individual circumstances and conditions.

HORMONAL CHANGES

Hormonal changes during perimenopause affect most of the tissue and organs in a woman's body. Reproductive organs, breasts, connective tissue in joints, skin, the urinary tract, liver, the cardiovascular system, and the central nervous system all have estrogen receptors. Fluctuations in hormones during perimenopause cause changes throughout the body that may or may not be noticeable for several years. Ovary function begins to decline in the mid-thirties, continues to decline at a faster rate in the forties, and stops in the late forties to early fifties.

The most common signs of the transition are hot flashes, night sweats, irregular menstrual periods, and vaginal dryness. Sleep disturbances are related mostly to hot flashes and night sweats. Interruptions in sleep can make fatigue, irritability, mood swings, and forgetfulness much worse. Vaginal dryness, urinary tract problems such as infections or incontinence, irritability, and mood swings can contribute to less interest in sex. Sexual interest is also influenced by the relationship a woman has with her partner as well as her own self-image as she experiences these changes in her body.

Changes in sexual function during perimenopause are not all related to the transition to menopause. Sexual health during midlife also is related to previous sexual health, attitudes, and experiences, as well as to general health. Women who have been sexually active before perimenopause tend to have fewer problems with vaginal dryness and atrophy, which are two of the major causes of sexual discomfort. Motivation and mood are important factors in whether a woman is interested in sex, and both may be affected during fluctuations in hormonal patterns. Having a regular sexual partner also influences a woman's interest and sexual health. In addition, during midlife both men and women may experience chronic disease such as diabetes, hypertension, and heart or breathing problems. These diseases and the side effects of medicines used to treat them also can affect motivation and mood.

Lillian's Story

Lillian had been having hot flashes, but they were not really bothering her too much. She thought she was handling the situation pretty well. Then night sweats became more bothersome, soaking her pajamas and sheets. That's when she decided to see her doctor.

I thought I could handle the changes, but when my night sweats were disturbing my husband's sleep, too, I felt I'd better do something about it. On my first visit for menopausal symptoms my doctor decided I wasn't menopausal. I don't know why, except he seemed to think I didn't "look" menopausal. Anyway, about six months later I tried again. This time he tested for hormone levels and told me I was in perimenopause. You know, after all that, I don't think it was the hot flashes that concerned me most. It was the vaginal dryness. It certainly affected my interest. I don't think I ever mentioned that to either my husband or my doctor. Looking back, I think I was embarrassed about it and must have thought it was a sign of getting old. I guess I'm just surprised at myself for falling for that old stereotype of the "menopausal woman." I didn't realize how powerful that image was in shaping my beliefs about myself, and mostly about my value as a person.

Part of society still regards midlife for a woman, and the aging process itself, as the beginning of the end—the end of sexual function and the end of life. It should be no surprise that many women feel powerless and disregarded at menopause. It is without doubt a time of change in roles and relationships in a woman's life, at home and at work, with children, partners, and parents, and in health related to chronic diseases. Yet, for many women, the end of the reproductive phase of their lives also can be positive. One obvious benefit is that once they are past perimenopause they are no longer bothered with the inconvenience, cramps, or premenstrual syndrome (PMS) that many women experience with monthly periods. Many women also enjoy an active sex life without having to worry about getting pregnant.

Cultural stereotypes of the aging woman are powerful influences on attitudes about perimenopausal symptoms. If hot flashes occur at work, some women may feel embarrassed and distracted, thinking their visible responses might compromise not only the quality of their work but also their regard by co-workers. Studies have linked low self-esteem with depression and feelings of helplessness in people who have chronic health problems. Although the transition to menopause is not a disease, it certainly is chronic, and for a disturbingly unspecified period of time. The added stress of not knowing when the next hot flash will occur increases distress. In bed, a woman may feel not only her own discomfort but the discomfort of her partner as well. For many women dealing · with these shared symptoms can add to self-doubt and negative feelings. A positive self-image helps maintain a balanced perspective. Of course, a healthy sense of humor helps too.

No scientific studies support the assumption that the transition to menopause causes such mental health problems as clinical depression, anxiety, or erratic behavior. Hormonal changes do contribute to mood swings. That these changes occur most notably during perimenopause has led to the assumption that fluctuating hormones are responsible for mental health problems. In fact, many other stresses a woman experiences at midlife can have a profound effect on mental health, and may be responsible for the rise in mood disorders that occurs during menopause. A depressed mood during perimenopause, as opposed to major or clinical depression, is intricately related to the status of older women in society, how women are treated at home and at work, and to other stress factors during midlife.

By the time a woman reaches her middle forties or fifties significant changes are occurring in many parts of her life. She may be facing the uncertainties of changing relations with family and friends. She may be trying to come to terms with the emotional, financial, and social aspects of divorce or the death of her partner. She may be caring for young children or adolescents living at home or returning home as young adults. She may be taking care of parents or in-laws, or dealing with the death or life-threatening illnesses of parents or friends. She may also be struggling with her own illnesses or changing expectations of career or education. Although men experience many of these life situations, women still tend to bear the major responsibility for the care of others. Given all these possibilites, it is not surprising that midlife women have physical and emotional symptoms, and sometimes feel overwhelmed.

SYMPTOMS

Researchers in North America and Europe have found that the symptoms women *expect* to have during perimenopause are based largely on cultural stereotypes and not necessarily on what most women experience. Women who have had problems with periods

(PMS) may be more likely to have perimenopausal symptoms and respond to those in similar ways, both physically and emotionally, than those without menstrual problems. It is interesting that fewer symptoms are reported in societies in which women can look forward to gaining social, religious, or political power after menopause. Different responses to perimenopause in other cultures also may be associated with diet, number of pregnancies, use of contraceptives, and physical activity.

Differences among women may be accounted for in part by the types and quality of studies done and which types of women were included in the studies. Early studies were conducted in Western cultures among white women of at least high school education who had talked with a medical professional about symptoms that were particularly bothersome or disruptive for them. However, among women surveyed in the Massachusetts Women's Health Study, only one-third of the women had actually talked with a physician about their symptoms (Leidy et al., 2000). Common medical beliefs about the menopausal woman clearly have been influenced by the experiences of those who have felt bad enough to seek medical care for their symptoms. Even so, interviews with large groups of women throughout the United States do show that many women experience fatigue, headache, irritability, and forgetfulness. However, the range and degree of symptoms are broad. For some women they are just an inconvenience. For others, they can be disabling.

Only 45 percent of women have hot flashes, and only 16.4 percent have night sweats. Irregular menstrual periods during the transition to menopause seem to be a problem for most women, and nearly as many feel a lack of energy. Periods can be longer or shorter, lighter or heavier, or just unpredictable. Some women also have stiff joints, difficulty concentrating, bloated stomach, decreased sexual drive, breast tenderness, and excessive bleeding.

Relief for hot flashes, sleep disturbances, and sexual discomforts can make a big difference in quality of life and self-image. Hot meals or drinks, hot weather or room temperature, or even too many blankets on the bed can make hot flashes worse. Wearing layers of clothing that can be removed if needed and using a fan both day and night can help. Staying away from too many sweets, high-fat meals, alcohol, and coffee, tea, or other drinks with caffeine can improve sleep. Exercising regularly also improves sleep. For discomfort during sexual intercourse, lubricating vaginal cream is helpful. Doing Kegel exercises regularly increases control if urine leakage is a problem during sex.

INTERPRETING MENOPAUSAL EXPERIENCES

By the year 2020, about 40 million women in America will be experiencing menopause. Yet it has been only a relatively short period of time that many physicians have paid attention to the individual changes associated with perimenopause. Despite more recent public attention about this natural life process, women who have perimenopausal symptoms still may be referred from specialist to specialist in search of treatment for what may seem to be elusive medical problems. Because each woman experiences perimenopause in her own way, it is possible that neither the woman nor her physician recognizes the symptoms. As a result many women may be either undertreated or overtreated for individual symptoms for months or even years. It can be frustrating and even frightening when physicians cannot find a cause, much less a "cure," for the symptoms. The added stress of not knowing what is happening can make symptoms worse.

One of the problems with diagnosing stages of menopause is that the signs and symptoms of perimenopause are not the same for every woman. There are hundreds of variations, and those differences alone defy the one-size-fits-all approach to treating menopause. Even more confounding to medical science, not to mention to women themselves, is that the way a woman feels about the changes at midlife is unique to her own emotional, psychological, and cultural experiences. Some women seem to breeze through the menopause years with only minor interruption to their lives. Others may feel nearly devastated by the experience. What causes such vast differences in an experience that is, biologically, a natural transition in a woman's life?

Menopause, just as other life phases, always embodies the whole of our life experiences. Each woman brings to midlife an interplay of biological function, responses to personal circumstances, and individual emotions. Some women feel completely out of control and victimized by their bodies. Others may prefer to think of menopause as a kind of dance, and marvel at the rituals and rhythms inherent in the process. Most women fit somewhere in the middle—sometimes feeling out of control and sometimes marveling at the wonder of it all.

Just as each woman experiences menopause in her own way, each also differs in the way she defines illness or seeks medical care for health problems. Women in particular are influenced by the experiences of family and friends. How women respond to the menopausal experience is also influenced by the way physicians regard and treat menopausal symptoms. Given conflicting messages about hormone replacement therapy as a cure-all, or the opposite extreme—"you'll just have to put up with it"—women must continually search for a rational middle ground.

Cultural and social factors also influence whether an individual seeks health care. Do we value traditional health care or do we rely on other treatments (herbs, supplements, or other over-the-counter remedies) for much of what ails us? Do we expect medicine to take care of all of the health problems we think we have? Do we think disease and disability are inevitable? Can we afford health care? (Lifestyle, not hormones, is the most significant factor affecting a woman's health in old age.) Still other factors include personality, education level, knowledge of the disease or condition, and preconceptions about the experience. For example, do we expect to have a horrible experience because our mother or someone else close to us had "the same thing" and really suffered because of it?

Women who have a poor self-image suffer more depression and distress during hot flashes and are more likely to feel unclean and embarrassed. Women who react more strongly to stress in their daily lives also tend to feel much more negatively about hot flashes. Personality differences influence the way we respond to the transition and to the medical language of menopause, such as *hormone deficiency disease* and *ovarian failure.* Instead, Gail Sheehy, author of *The Silent Passage* (1998), proposes the more positive term, *ovarian fulfillment.* Women who view menopause as a medical problem tend to have a more difficult experience and are frustrated because no straightforward cure exists. For these women menopause can be a negative symbol of aging, not a journey into the wise-woman years, but a rapid decline toward irretrievable loss.

Where do women find hope in the transition through menopause? From the 1960s to the 1990s the most prevalent images of menopausal women in medical literature were physical deterioration, psychological disability, and social worthlessness. It is not a pretty picture, and it does not reflect the experiences of most women. More women today are seeking answers, support, and an expanded community with whom to share their concerns and ways to cope. Although no single menopause experience applies to every woman, most can feel less uncertain or fearful by sharing experiences and learning from others who are going through it. It may be surprising to learn how positive others feel, even with hot flashes (power surges!), and how fulfilling their own lives can be, enriched by the self-knowledge gained from integrating the emotional, physical, and spiritual elements of their lives during midlife.

A bountiful source of hope can be the stories of women who are in their postmenopausal years. I (JH) know a group of women, now in their early sixties, who gathered together recently for a high school girlfriends reunion. Most had not had contact for more than forty years, until the need to connect to old friendships drew them from different parts of the country to a mountain cabin similar to the one they had visited from time to time as teenagers. On the first night they sat around the fireplace and began to tell their stories. They had lived through good and bad marriages, life-threatening diseases, the painful and often prolonged development of children into adulthood, raising their children and sometimes their grandchildren, and the death of family members and friends. They had worked to pay bills and worked for the love of it. They had led lives they could never have predicted as young adults.

Throughout the telling, and throughout the following days, they laughed and cried and planned the next time they would be together. As for menopause, by that time it had become just a footnote marking their early middle years, only a small part of all the experiences that shaped their lives. For women just entering the transition to menopause, and feeling nearly overwhelmed by it, this perspective carries a strong message of hope.

Chapter 2

Closing and Opening Doors: Dealing with a Journey of Personal Loss

When one door closes, another door opens.

TRANSITIONS DURING MENOPAUSE

Menopause encompasses many transitions, and the journey occurs over the span of several years. During this time in a woman's life menopause often brings a sense of uncertainty, change, and an underlying sense of loss. The social and personal meaning of menopause varies greatly among women, but its significance can be noted in the oft-repeated phrase "change of life." Socially, the significance of menopause is influenced directly by the culture in which a woman lives. On a more personal level, many women see it as a milestone, a rite of passage, and an important phase in the developmental life cycle. With this milestone many women feel as if doors are closing on important parts of their life such as child-bearing and child rearing, a youthful body, and monthly menstrual cycles. At the same time many women also see menopause as the opening of another door, with new perspectives, lifestyle changes, and new goals. It is this positive view that is associated with better health and fewer symptoms in menopause.

Whether the door is opening or closing, many women view menopause as a series of journeys through doors of uncertainty. Basically, the midlife can be broken down into three separate journeys: physical, spiritual, and interpersonal. It includes internal and external doors. It is a time when women reflect on what life has given them and turn to the door in front of them to see what might lie ahead.

In midlife and menopause a woman's physical body undergoes a journey involving mystery, loss, and struggle. Women often fear hot flashes, mood swings, and physical changes in the body when entering menopause. What was once a predictable rhythm of monthly cycles suddenly becomes unpredictable. Menstrual bleeding may often increase, become heavier and more irregular, and ultimately stop. What was once a svelte physique slowly begins to sag and change its appearance. Some women see the changes as the end of a beautiful physical body, whereas others see them as an opportunity to have a healthier body and lifestyle. Some women find the changes minor and function well throughout menopause. Others experience changes during menopause that they find disabling. Women's reactions to the physical changes are highly variable and often dependent on a woman's cultural status and preconceived notions about menopause itself.

A woman's spiritual journey during midlife is often the most significant of the three journeys. During this time women often feel the need to address who they are outside of traditional roles of mother, wife, and daughter. Priorities are often redefined, and women often use midlife as a time to become the person they want to be. The doors of childbearing, child rearing, and career building are often closed by midlife, and many menopausal women seek ways to open doors to new experiences. In addition, women who are dealing with their own mortality often deepen their spiritual links with organized religion.

From an interpersonal standpoint, women in midlife seek new paths in relationships with their children, life partners, aging parents or relatives, and careers. As these changing relationships evolve a certain amount of struggle and loss occurs. Parenting roles often change as children enter adolescence and young adulthood. The doors of parental responsibilities begin to close, creating newfound time to devote to relationships with spouses or life partners. It is also during this time that women feel the increased responsibilities of caring for aging relatives—reversing roles of child and caretaker.

Regardless of perspective, menopause offers women an opportunity to look at themselves, and challenges them to open new doors to spiritual and personal growth.

PHYSICAL AND SOCIAL CONTEXT OF MENOPAUSE

FM is a sixty-five-year-old woman who eagerly shared her reflections about menopause.

When I was in my forties I was still busy raising my two teenagers, keeping up with my household responsibilities, and helping my husband run our private pharmacy. Menopause sort of sneaked up on me—it began as sporadic periods over several months to a year. My periods were unpredictable and seemed to last several days longer than normal. All of a sudden, I felt sad when I realized that my family was probably complete, whether I liked it or not. I mourned silently for a few months since there would be no more babies to cuddle. Oh well, I didn't need to worry about getting pregnant anymore, so all those pills and condoms were a thing of the past!

One summer when I was in my mid-forties, I donned my bathing suit for the beach. As I stood in front of the full-length mirror in my bedroom, I noticed my first gray hairs, my flabby arms, the so-called "chicken neck" with all those wrinkles, and those unsightly varicose veins bulging out like the eyes on a frog. My boobs weren't so perky either. Oh well, there was nothing there that a good hairdresser and a great plastic surgeon couldn't spruce up. Besides, my kids were practically grown—there was no excuse I could use to postpone a much-needed exercise program. At my last checkup my doctor had urged me to exercise regularly to get in shape. And then, those dreadful hot flashes! They felt more like power surges that jolted me awake at night. My doctor insisted that all I needed was "Vitamin P"—Prempro. I tried it for a while but stopped because I felt bloated all the time and gained weight. Eventually the hot flashes stopped, and now I love not having a period. For once, the only pads and tampons I purchased were for my teenage daughter. Finally I've come to the realization that menopause really is the change of life that my own mother had called it. It changed my whole perspective on life. I have realized that I have accomplished much in my life, both before and after menopause. There may not be any more children of my own, but I have high hopes for the children that I do have. I don't sweat the small stuff anymore. Rather, I savor each new day as an opportunity to be better—a better person, a better wife, and a better mother.

Similar to FM's story, life in general presents a continuum of transitions. Uniquely, though, menopause often presents challenges not seen in the rest of the life cycle. In the book *Transformation Through Menopause,* Marian Van Eyk McCain (1991) presents menopause as an overlapping and simultaneous set of transitions. During menopause, certain life events are shaped by changing relationships with children, spouses, and family members, health concerns, and interpersonal changes. In explaining women's reactions to all these changes, McCain proposes four major themes of menopause.

The first theme, "biology is destiny," focuses on a woman's loss of childbearing abilities. This end of fertility represents a loss, and women's reactions to this loss are highly variable. For some the end of fertility is a welcome relief leading to the door of increased sexual freedom. For others, though, this loss of fertility is a closed door that cannot be reentered. It is a time that seems particularly final for those who have chosen not to have children or who have experienced the loss of a child. Regardless of this difference in reaction, McCain feels that menopause creates the necessity for women to redefine themselves as more than just bearers of children.

McCain's second theme, "fading roses," takes into account the changes in physical status and appearance that are part of aging. The reflection in the mirror now shows gray hair, dry skin, wrinkles, and sagging breasts. In a society that values youth and the "perfect" body, confronting these physical changes can be seen as a closed door, affecting a woman's self-esteem and sexuality. Not all women, though, are defined by their physical appearance. For up to 75 percent of women menopause presents an opportunity to be healthier and make considerable changes in their personal lifestyle.

The third theme, "medicalization of menopause," refers to the process by which medical providers (physicians, pharmaceutical companies) define menopause as a medical condition that needs to be treated. This medicalization process can be construed as taking natural human life cycles and creating medical problems of them. The use of hormone replacement therapy as a treatment for menopause is a prime example of this. More recently, women have sought to use more natural and homeopathic products to ease the physical discomforts of menopause. Many want to avoid prescription medications and reject the medicalization of this life event.

The last theme identified by McCain is "rehearsal for death." Included in each of the smaller transitions of menopause are a series of little deaths, or closing doors. These transitions are the end of fertility, loss of natural hormones, and fading physical appearance. This theme represents the death of parts of the familiar self women have lived with their entire lives. As described, this "rehearsal" gives women an opportunity to reflect on their own mortality and the inevitability of death.

THE SPIRITUAL ISSUES

No matter a woman's cultural background, her personal spirituality affects her views of herself and the world around her. More broadly, spirituality can be defined as beliefs that give transcendent meaning to one's life. Menopause is a time that forces a woman to pause, to look at how her own beliefs have shaped the person she has become and perhaps the woman she would like to be.

Julie recently reflected on her perimenopause experience: "I was just starting to miss periods occasionally and get whiffs of hot flashes. Then came the dreaded report—my mammogram was abnormal! The biopsy proved the worst and I soon found myself undergoing lumpectomy surgery, not once, but twice, then total mastectomy and breast reconstruction. God and the prayers of my friends and family have kept me going. I try to look at things positively, with hope. My plastic surgeon said he was just 'an instrument of God.'

"I was looking at myself in the mirror today, two weeks after the breast reconstruction. My tummy is flatter where they removed tissue to remake my left breast, and my new left breast is bigger than before.

After chemotherapy, the plastic surgeon says he can insert an implant into the right breast to make it the same size as my new left one. I will look better than before! Yes, I have lost a breast, my periods will be gone soon after chemotherapy starts, and I will lose my hair, but I have had uplifting and spiritual support like I never knew before. My friend said she had a vision of a guardian angel enveloping me. I have been able to share my faith with many people at the hospital. I have a peace in my heart that everything is going to be okay."

Menopause brings many changes in perspective, including spiritual perspective. It is when many women ask Why am I here? and What am I here for? Women are often more spiritual and more religiously active than men. Perhaps as a result, women may be more likely to use their spiritual resources when faced with a crisis, as did Julie. She faced the challenge of having breast cancer with the added benefit of spiritual resources such as prayer and religious involvement in addition to her personal resources. I (DK) remember seeing the large basket of cards in her room one day, and I remarked that she was going to need a bigger basket. Her confidence and hope were evident to everyone she encountered.

Women who want to explore further the spiritual aspects of purpose may find the book *The Purpose-Driven Life: What on Earth Am I Here For?* (2002), by Rick Warren, an excellent resource. In his book he addresses the question What on earth am I here for? from the spiritual perspective. He addresses the issue of purpose from a very practical, sometimes humorous, and distinctly biblical view. Women such as Julie who rely on spiritual strength when facing serious issues in the midlife may find great solace in the book.

THE INTERPERSONAL CHANGES

MW is a fifty-four-year-old woman who recently described her personal entry into menopause as somewhat stressful.

All of a sudden, I looked around and everything had changed. My children were all grown. My daughter was married and expecting her first child. My son was single, but well on his way to a successful career as a lawyer. I think what stopped me in my tracks was the quiet—the stillness in the house that was deafening at times. All at once, there were no baseball or football games to attend, no endless dance recitals, no parent-teacher conferences, and no one to tuck into bed at night. What was I supposed to do? How could I possibly occupy all my free time that stood endlessly before me? Then I realized the day had come that I had waited for so long. I could choose to do what I wanted to do for myself and for others. My husband and I could discuss the day's events without an impatient interruption. We could go to dinner anywhere we pleased and not worry about a babysitter. Over time I began to deepen friendships with women with whom I had once shared babysitters. We had lunch together, played golf together, and showed off pictures of "Grandma's kids" to each other. We shared all the menopause jokes and remedies for the "flashes." More importantly, I found time for just *me* . . . eating right, exercising more, and splurging on a new outfit instead of shoes for the children. Finally, I could embrace my passion—painting with oils. I even donated one of my seascape paintings to a local children's charity for their annual auction last summer.

As children grow up and enter adolescence and young adulthood, a woman's role becomes one of launching children. As children become more independent, another door closes for their mother. For women who have devoted much of their time to child care and childbearing, this empty nest often brings with it increased risk of developing depression. Other women may view child launching as a relief and see it as an opportunity for new freedom and devoting more time to themselves and their communities.

Once child rearing is complete, men often begin to focus more on the family whereas generally women focus on work and community commitments. This time is obviously a major life shift in a couples' relationship. As much as 11 percent of divorces occur in couples married twenty years or more. Just as many women begin to make headway in their careers and enjoy new freedom from child rearing, many also begin to deal with caring for older relatives. Even with married couples the primary role of caretaker for aging parents and in-laws often falls to the woman. The role reversal that occurs between aging relatives and their adult children presents another challenge. The elderly often feel a loss of control, and the midlife woman may feel a loss of parents as role models and as a strong, dependable part of her life.

Grandchildren offer another significant change in family dynamics. Happily, as the role of responsibility as a parent lessens, the opportunity for being a fun-loving grandparent presents itself. Grandparents may feel some doors closing on their own lives but find doors open to the joy of sharing family history and traditions that grandchildren can carry into the future.

OPENING DOORS FOR OTHERS

Women's attitudes about their menopausal experience have become more open in the 1990s. Information about menopause is also more available in books and magazines and through the Internet. Women also are often involved in support networks of women experiencing similar life events, and those who have gone before can lead the way in opening new doors for others. In the bittersweet experience of menopause women have both losses and gains, and can be empowered to become more capable and courageous in facing what lies ahead, after "the change."

Powerful insights on the open-door perspective can be heard in the words of the following reflections of a friend:

I think of the word *menopause* as having a lot of meanings, and a lot of them have been negative. Society definitely emphasizes that there clearly is a loss. On one level there is quite a loss and grieving that comes with one's body changing . . . and a lot of lost aspirations and ideals. But there are many more good feelings and experiences. The greatest of these is the recognition that I have come a long way on life's journey. It gives me pause to reflect not only on the wisdom I have gained from where I have been, but on the opportunities for personal growth and sharing with others that will come in the future.

Chapter 3

Mood and the Mind in Menopause

INTRODUCTION

In a society that places so much emphasis on youth and being mentally quick, menopause must seem as if it is the beginning of the end. Some of the early symptoms of menopause may be very subtle, such as forgetting your best friend's birthday, unexpected momentary memory blanks, feeling mentally fuzzy, waves of warmness, and feeling just a little irritated at the young, attractive female waitress that served you dinner in a local restaurant. It may seem as if Alzheimer's disease is setting in, but it could just be the beginning of menopause. Feelings of depression sometimes occur, followed by a loss of interest in activities. Are these symptoms normal menopause, or do they signal depression? The following story illustrates the dilemma that many menopausal women live with every day.

Anne's Story

Anne was forty-eight when she found out that she had breast cancer. She had been having frequent hot flashes, had stopped having periods a little more than a year before, and was still dealing with the fact that her children were no longer living at home. One child was in college, one was getting married, and now she was faced with the news that she had breast cancer. Cancer! It was almost too much to bear. She wrestled with images of her changed body, of losing her breast, and the fear of not being a woman anymore. Some days she felt like crying, other days she seemed to find the strength to overcome her sadness. She was anxious, sweaty, and didn't sleep well at times. Was this normal?

Now her doctor was asking her to make decisions she did not feel ready to make, no matter how many times he explained the choices. How extensive did the surgery need to be? Should she go ahead with plastic surgery to reconstruct her breast? Could the family afford that? Where could she turn for help with her decisions? Although she considered medical knowledge and skill most important in a physician, she also wanted her doctor to understand her need to deal with the practical and emotional questions as well as the medical issues she was facing.

Many potential issues converge to bring enormous stress on the menopausal woman: physical changes, emotional stress, medical illness, and psychological and sexual health. Hot flashes, the end of the menstrual cycle, and sleep disturbances are the symptoms that often get the most press. Some of the most important and often overlooked issues are the psychological challenges that collide during menopause. Apprehension, mood swings, feelings of grief, and family change often travel hand in hand during the menopause journey. They can be much worse when a woman also faces a serious illness. Anxiety may have many sources, including lack of knowledge about physical changes, sexual changes, mood swings, uncertainties in dealing with difficult life decisions, or a true anxiety disorder. Most women who go through menopause are not physically ill but may have difficult periods of self-doubt and confusion. The physical effects of menopause are compounded by the aging effects of midlife, a sense of loss that accompanies the empty-nest syndrome, and social changes. How much these psychological changes are the result of hormonal changes is still the subject of intense debate.

ATTITUDES TOWARD THE MENOPAUSE TRANSITION

Even if the medical community labels menopause as an illness in search of hormones, women tend to view menopause as merely a life event, or a rite of passage. More than half of women refer to menopause as just the end of menstruation, and a little more than a third view menopause as an end to childbearing potential. A survey of women who took part in the Seattle Midlife Women's Health Study found similar attitudes: women viewed menopause as a normal developmental process (Woods and Mitchell, 1999). In fact, most of the uncertainty women express about menopause relates to their own expectations of menopause itself. The largest study of menopausal women, the North American Menopause Society survey, conducted in 1994, found the majority of women see menopause and midlife as the beginning of positive life and health changes. For example, more than 75 percent of women said they had made health-related lifestyle changes such as quitting smoking at menopause.

Menopause represents a developmental stage in the life cycle and a change in the status of the "nest" or home environment and relationships. During this stage, women gradually adjust to social, psychological, and spiritual changes that accompany recognized symptoms and physical changes. Along with the physical changes, significant psychological events also occur during midlife. Some of these events include changing relationships with children. As children grow up both physically and mentally—leaving the nest for college, jobs, marriage, or parenthood—some women may feel a sense of tremendous loss and grief.

Midlife and menopause also bring changing relationships with a spouse or significant other. Relationships can undergo tremendous instability once children have left home. Couples often need to redefine their relationship as children begin to be less of a day-to-day priority.

Not all women, however, find their nest empty in menopause. More women are extending or beginning their childbearing years well into their forties, often with the help of in vitro fertilization. These women have full nests and find young toddlers and children at home at the same time they are dealing with fatigue, irritability, and the physical symptoms of menopause. As a result of parenting well into the menopausal years, many women may feel out of place as they try to fit in with the younger parents of their children's peer group.

On the other end of the child-adult spectrum, menopause and the midlife time may also bring the serious illness or loss of one's parents. These loved ones often need additional help or supervision of their care, stretching the reserves of energy, time, and financial resources of their adult children. They may even move into the homes of their adult children. This added burden can cause emotional stress in addition to physical exhaustion, and may trigger depression or serious illness in midlife women.

SOCIAL CHANGES AND CONTEXT OF MENOPAUSE

Women have different expectations of menopause, and cultural background may have significant influence on a woman's response to menopause. This reaction is often affected by a woman's status in her own culture—whether she is valued or devalued. Women who define themselves primarily in a childbearing role seem to experience the most distress. Studies show that women cope with menopause differently within different cultures. In cultures in which women are given more status when they are beyond child-bearing years, or in which menopause is viewed more as a normal life stage, women seem to have fewer problems with it.

Unfortunately, women in the United States tend to be valued in terms of youth and sexual attractiveness and often are considered less "valuable" as they age. Women in the workplace also face conflicting roles as mother, spouse, and breadwinner, and feel that they are punished for responsibilities outside the workplace. Concerns about sexual harassment, unequal pay, and fewer opportunities than available to male co-workers also increase the risk of depression and anxiety. These concerns contribute to feelings that menopause is a negative experience. However, a wider variety of choices, including educational and career opportunities, delayed or forgone childbearing, and single-parenting options, have helped lessen emphasis on more traditional views of women's roles in the family and society.

Women in some other cultures have different experiences. For example, Japanese women seem to have significantly fewer hot flashes than women in North America and Europe. Except for irregular periods, Mayan women report essentially no menopausal symptoms. Although cultural perceptions of menopause may change the way a woman feels about physical changes and symptoms, differences in lifestyle and diet during menopause also may play a part.

DOES MENOPAUSE CAUSE DEPRESSION?

Depression is more than a bad mood or the "blues"; it is a serious medical illness that affects women's physical as well as mental health. Menopause and depression occur simultaneously in many women, but menopause does not cause depression. Depression is twice as frequent in women compared to men, and is common among women at the midlife. Many theories have been suggested to explain why depression occurs more frequently in women. There seems some biochemical support for the role that hormones play in the development of mood disorders such as anxiety or depression. A well-recognized fork in the road begins in adolescence—a splitting of the incidence of depression between men and women. This gender difference begins in the teenage years and ends at midlife, after which rates of depression gradually rise and become higher in men. Hormones such as estrogen and progesterone have an effect on the brain chemicals that are associated with mood. Women may also experience other mood-related disorders linked to the menstrual cycle or pregnancy, including premenstrual syndrome and postpartum depression. Women who have experienced premenstrual syndrome have a higher incidence of depression. Depression also has been associated with hormonal medications such as birth control pills, especially in women over age thirty-five.

Some research studies have linked estrogen and hormonal treatment to improvements in thinking processes and the possibility of preventing and treating depression. Researchers have still not completely sorted out what role, if any, hormonal treatment might have in treating depression or anxiety. Some studies say that it helps, while others say it makes no difference. It is known that antidepressants work well in most cases. Women who are depressed should seek medical attention immediately. It is important to know that good treatment is available and that medications have minimal side effects. Counseling also can be very helpful. (Chapter 4 has more information about the types of counseling available and which one might be appropriate for you.)

Early results of the Study of Women's Health by the National Institutes on Aging seem to show that African-American women have more estrogen-related symptoms at menopause, and Asian women report less severe menopausal symptoms than white or African-American women (Fitzpatrick and Santen, 2002). Factors related to mood at menopause include depression or PMS before menopause, hysterectomy, emotional or family stress, a negative attitude toward menopause, and poor health and lifestyle choices such as smoking and lack of exercise.

Risk Factors for Depression

Social and psychological factors also play a role in the development of depression; for example, happily married women have lower rates of major depression than single women. Common risk

---

EXHIBIT 3.1. Common Risk Factors for Depression

- Childhood loss, such as a death or prolonged illness of parent or sibling
- Low self-esteem
- Lower socioeconomic levels
- Family history of depression
- Physical or sexual abuse as child or adult
- Lower educational level
- Stress from multiple roles in family (spouse, mother, home, work responsibility)
- Marital stress
- Recent birth of a child
- Body scars or disfigurement from trauma or surgery
- Female gender
- Children in home with attention deficit disorders
- Recent pregnancy loss or abortion

Source: Adapted from Huston JE and Lanka LD (1997). *Perimenopause: Changes in Women's Health after 35.* Oakland, CA: New Harbinger Publications, Inc.

factors for depression are listed in Exhibit 3.1. Women with these factors should pay special attention to the symptoms of depression. Spouses and other loved ones need to be understanding and supportive in getting help when it is needed.

The symptoms of depression are listed in Exhibit 3.2. The first two symptoms are the most important. A sad mood is expected in someone with depression but may not always be evident. Many women will appear calm and pleasant even when they are suffering immensely on the inside. In our medical practice we often see women who have managed to hide their sadness for a long time. When the dam finally breaks it can be a painful and emotional experience. It takes emotional strength for depressed women to finally seek help. We urge women to see a physician sooner rather than later, because treatment is available and is almost always effective.

The second symptom is loss of interest in activities. This can happen at any life stage, but it can be more troublesome at midlife. Women at this stage of life are usually very busy with work and home obligations, responsibilities for teenaged children, and other activities. When women with such great responsibilities begin to

---

EXHIBIT 3.2. Symptoms of Depression

- Persistent sad, anxious, or "empty" mood
- Loss of interest or pleasure in hobbies and activities that were once enjoyed, including sex
- Feelings of hopelessness, pessimism
- Feelings of guilt, worthlessness, helplessness
- Decreased energy; fatigue; being "slowed down"
- Difficulty concentrating, remembering, making decisions
- Insomnia, early-morning awakening, oversleeping
- Appetite and/or weight loss or overeating and weight gain
- Thoughts of death or suicide; suicide attempts
- Restlessness, irritability
- Persistent physical symptoms that do not respond to treatment such as headaches, digestive disorders, and chronic pain

Source: From the National Institute of Mental Health, "What Every Woman Should Know," <www.nimh.nih.gov/publicat/depwomenknows.cfm>, accessed October 22, 2003.

pull back and stop participating the effects are felt throughout the family. Because of women's central role at home, a lack of interest in activities can have a profound effect on husbands, children, co-workers, and others. Loved ones who see this happening must help the woman seek medical help before a crisis occurs. If she is not convinced she needs help, try to convince her to take an online screening test, available at <www.depression-screening.org>, which is sponsored by the National Mental Health Association. This simple, confidential test can be taken in the privacy of the home or at any public library computer with Internet capability.

The other symptoms listed are present to varying degrees in women with depression. Depression shows itself differently in every person. Poor appetite, poor sleep, and persistent physical symptoms are particularly common symptoms in midlife women. Women with these symptoms should seek medical attention even if they have no persistent changes in mood, since the appetite and sleep disturbances may be the first signs, and the depressed mood may come later. Because lack of sleep and weight loss can cause other medical problems, seeking treatment should not be delayed.

The symptom of suicidal thoughts deserves special mention. Such thoughts are not considered unusual in depressed women, especially if they are fleeting. However, persistent thoughts of suicide and severe emotional states, along with alcohol or drug use, or specific methods and plans for suicide are *emergency* warnings that need to be addressed on an *urgent* basis. Call your local crisis hotline or the emergency department of your local hospital for guidance. Always take suicide thoughts seriously. Life is precious, and more people care than you may realize.

SPIRITUALITY AND DEPRESSION

Depression affects more than 10 million women in the United States each year. That number alone is reason enough to explore every avenue of support and assistance, including spiritual and religious resources. A considerable amount of research on the role of spiritual factors in mental illness has focused on depression, and has shown that a person who incorporates religion and spirituality in his or her treatment typically has fewer symptoms of depression. If women are depressed, strong spiritual support can help in the recovery process.

Treatment of depression is enhanced when religious and spiritual factors are taken into account. Therapy that is sensitive to a woman's spiritual and religious context is at least equal to and often superior to standard treatment. Some women may prefer to seek counseling from certified pastoral counselors/therapists who have received training in both the traditional counseling and religious disciplines.

ANXIETY DISORDERS

As with depression, symptoms of anxiety may increase just before menopause, but no evidence supports menopause as a specific cause of anxiety disorders. Still, as with depression, women suffer from anxiety disorders at twice the rate of men. One of the most common types of anxiety disorder is panic disorder. Women with this disorder have feelings of anxiety and terror that strike suddenly and repeatedly with no warning. They are unable to predict when an attack will occur. Many develop intense anxiety between episodes, worrying when and where the next one will strike.

The symptoms of a panic attack include pounding heart, sweating, and feeling weak, faint, or dizzy. Tingling in the hands or numbness may occur in addition to feeling flushed or chilled. These feelings may be accompanied by chest pains or smothering sensations, nausea, and a fear of impending doom. Many women have expressed that it felt as if they were going to have a heart attack, or were losing their mind, or were even dying. Panic attacks can occur at any time, even during sleep. An attack generally peaks within ten minutes, but some symptoms may last longer.

Treatment usually involves both medications and psychotherapy. Common medications used include selective serotonin reuptake inhibitors (SSRIs). These medications act in the brain on a chemical messenger called serotonin. SSRIs are commonly used because they tend to have fewer side effects than older antidepressants. It may be confusing that a doctor may prescribe antidepressant medications for anxiety, but many of the SSRIs also are effective treatment for anxiety disorders. Other medications used to treat anxiety disorders include monoamine oxidase (MAO) inhibitors, tricyclic medications, azipirones, and benzodiazepines. However, all of these are used less commonly than SSRIs because they have more frequent side effects or are not as effective for some women. In addition, benzodiazepines (such as Valium) can be habit forming and may not be best for long-term use. Some women have withdrawal symptoms when they stop taking benzodiazepines, and the symptoms of anxiety can return after the medications are stopped.

Psychotherapy is effective for several anxiety disorders, particularly panic disorder and social phobia. Termed *cognitive-behavioral therapy,* the treatment requires regular visits to a qualified therapist for twelve weeks or longer. The therapy aims to reframe a patient's point of view toward his or her phobias and fears and deal with specific behaviors that need to be changed. A combination of medication and psychotherapy is the best approach for many women.

CHANGES IN SEXUALITY

If the role of hormones regarding depression seems unclear, the picture regarding changes in female sexuality with menopause is even fuzzier. Sexual problems are common for women in midlife. Because of menopausal symptoms, woman are more likely than men to seek physical and mental health care and are more likely to suffer from depression and other psychiatric diseases. Problems have been common in research studies looking at sexuality in menopause. Most studies have not taken into account sexual difficulties before menopause, other causes of stress, the health status of partners, or psychiatric illness not at all related to menopausal symptoms. As well, it is hard to define sexual dysfunction. It is a relative term, often related more to satisfaction with the relationship than to a particular physical cause. Sexual desire decreases with age, and the frequency of sexual activity and orgasm also decreases. It is unclear, though, whether menopause truly causes these changes. Some studies have found little effect of menopausal status (including decreasing levels of estrogen and testosterone) on sexual function, with most of the menopausal effects being a small reduction in sexual enjoyment and sex drive. Libido and frequency of sexual activity and orgasm may decrease during the transition to menopause; however, satisfaction with the sexual relationship is largely unaffected for most women. In fact, many women feel that menopause brings sexual freedom—a freedom from birth control and fear of pregnancy.

Do I Need Viagra?

Some women seem to be able to increase their sex drive with medications that contain testosterone. Side effects, though, may be troublesome, and include increased hair growth on the face and body. For many women, testosterone treatment may not be any more effective than the testosterone a woman's body produces naturally. The decrease in estrogen production during perimenopause is much greater than the decrease in testosterone. The effect is that there is a relatively greater proportion of testosterone to estrogen than before perimenopause. That could have a positive effect on sexual desire, along with the more assertive behavior we see in many women at midlife. Although Viagra may be seen as the "magic bullet" for men's sexual dysfunction, no studies yet prove that Viagra plays a positive role in a woman's sexual interest or satisfaction.

MENOPAUSE TREATMENT ISSUES

Counseling and medications have a role in assisting women facing the psychological challenges and physical symptoms of menopause. Hormone replacement has been used to help alleviate some physical symptoms. Treatment for psychological issues in menopause may include prescription medication, herbal remedies, exercise, and/or counseling. Estrogen may moderate mood swings to a limited degree, but for many women it has limited direct effect on mood. Because the role of estrogen is not well defined, and proven treatment is available, depression is best treated with antidepressants and psychotherapy, as discussed previously. Anxiety should be treated with medication and/or psychotherapy as well.

Exercise is highly recommended for menopausal women as an effective self-treatment for anxiety and depression, along with medical treatment and counseling if they are recommended by a doctor. Moderate physical activity for as little as three hours a week can benefit overall health, and many women find it can also reduce symptoms of depression.

Counseling is an important therapy for a variety of psychological symptoms and conditions in menopause and is useful for helping women in the transition into menopause. Women do not need to be depressed or have an "official" anxiety disorder in order to benefit from counseling. Counseling also is beneficial for women who are having marital conflict as a result of mood swings or other stresses. Marriage and family therapists have specific training to assist women with marital issues and are often sensitive to spiritual issues that may accompany marital conflict. Counseling is helpful also for specific anxiety disorders and depression, alone or in combination with medication. Brief office counseling from a family physician often helps, especially if a woman is reluctant to visit a psychiatrist or is afraid of being labeled as having a mental health problem. Often it is a huge relief just to know the difference between normal symptoms during menopause and true illness, and the family physician can often assist in this process. When serious depression or anxiety disorders are found, the family doctor can provide treatment directly, or, more often, provide treatment in partnership with other mental health providers such as psychiatrists and therapists.

Where can women find hope in the many challenging and stressful moods of menopause and the midlife? Knowing what to expect in menopause, the role of hormones, and which treatments are available may help prevent depression and anxiety and encourage women to seek early treatment. Women who know the signs and symptoms of serious anxiety or depressive illness will be best prepared to prevent further problems, and will be better able to get themselves back on track.

Chapter 4

Counseling and Group Support

Oh yes, I am wise, but it's wisdom born of pain,
Yes, I've paid the price, but look how much I've gained!

Helen Reddy, "I Am Woman"

SEEKING COUNSELING

Counseling can be an important part of therapy for a variety of psychological symptoms and conditions during menopause. It can be extremely useful in making the transition through menopause much easier. Understanding normal symptoms of menopause and common psychological concerns can be very reassuring. Relief often comes from just knowing that other women have similar symptoms and distress.

When a woman is concerned about menopause she should first talk with her family physician or gynecologist for counseling and education. If the problems extend beyond usual menopause symptoms the physician may refer the woman to a psychiatrist, a clinical psychologist, a marriage and family therapist, or a pastoral counselor. Many types of therapists are available.

Rita had to admit things were getting out of control. Her periods had stopped, she was having headaches, and she could not sleep due to hot flashes. She was irritable, and her teenaged daughter had recently started talking about having sex! How was she supposed to remain coherent during a discussion about abstinence, condoms, and sexually transmitted diseases when her head was pounding? To top it all off, she and her husband Rick were not getting along. He was always wanting to go fishing and hardly ever stayed home on the weekends. He would leave Saturday at 4 a.m. and not come home until Sunday afternoon. Was she supposed to raise the kids by herself?

She went to her doctor for her annual exam. The doctor noticed that Rita was not her usual self. After asking her several questions, her doctor said she needed to learn to handle stress better, and that she might be depressed. The doctor recommended that she see a psychologist. "Me, see a psychologist?" thought Rita. "What will people think?" She never dreamed she would have to seek formal counseling. She definitely would have to think about it before agreeing to see a psychologist.

Rita's situation shows the difficulty many women have in accepting that they may need formal counseling help. The whole idea of therapy sounds scary. Women do not want to be labeled as "crazy," and fear that seeing a counselor or therapist will somehow brand them. The fact is, counseling is extremely valuable for many women. After the initial resistance most women see that psychological counseling is beneficial and not as scary as they once thought. They are also reassured by knowing that counseling is private and confidential. This fact helps overcome the initial reluctance to open up and tell a counselor one's true feelings. It also helps overcome the initial reluctance to participate in therapy. Conversations and medical records are protected by law and cannot be seen by anyone, including a spouse, without the permission of the person receiving therapy. Rita, after learning that her privacy would be protected, and after meeting the psychologist and finding out she was warm and understanding, returned for several counseling visits and eventually improved greatly.

INDIVIDUAL COUNSELING

How can a woman find the kind of help she needs? Finding a therapist is not like choosing a plumber—asking a friend or looking in the phone book may not be the best approach. When a woman needs help with serious behavioral or mental health issues she wants to have a voice in the selection of the counselor. Counseling is personal, private, and intimate. The person she chooses may hear more about her feelings than her close friends or even her mate. One should have realistic expectations, since counselors and therapists are not superpeople, and women should understand the basic approach(es) the therapist plans to use ("What do you mean you plan to *hypnotize* me?") so that there are fewer surprises. As well, one should not give up at the first sign of conflict. Counseling is likely to touch on some very sensitive issues. So how does a woman choose someone to hear her most private and intimate feelings, and listen while she wrestles with some of the biggest issues she has ever had to face?

Asking the family physician or gynecologist for advice is an excellent first step. Depending on the individual difficulty or issue, the doctor will have specific recommendations. Therapists often specialize and develop expertise in certain fields just as medical specialists do. Thus, the physician might recommend one person for dealing with depression, another if the problem is stress, or another if the need is for marriage counseling.

Counselors/therapists have different types of training, skills, and experience. Knowing more about the types of counselors most often needed by women at midlife will help in selecting the right therapist. Is the therapist a doctor? Has the counselor had experience with women who have had similar problems? Is the therapist likely to take spiritual background into account? Will he or she recommend medications, or therapy alone?

TYPES OF THERAPISTS

Marriage and Family Therapists

Marriage and family therapists are licensed mental health professionals trained in psychotherapy and family systems. They treat people within the context of marriage, couple relationships, and family systems. Typically, marriage and family therapists go beyond the traditional emphasis on the individual to attend to the nature and role of individuals in the context of the marriage and the family. They are concerned with the overall, long-term well-being of individuals and their families, and often include the patient's spiritual and religious perspective in counseling. Marriage and family therapists have graduate training, either a master's degree or doctoral degree (PhD), and at least two years of clinical experience before they begin practice. They do not prescribe medications themselves, and often work in partnership with other physicians or therapists, although they can work alone.

Clinical Psychologists

Clinical psychologists are licensed and usually have a doctoral degree in the study of the human mind and human behavior. They may work in many different settings, including hospitals, clinics, schools, and private offices. In addition to helping people deal with stress and mental health issues such as anxiety and depression, many also help treat patients with spinal cord injuries, chronic pain or illness, stroke, arthritis, or neurologic conditions. Their diverse training also prepares them to work with women who are dealing a variety of issues, including depression, personal crises, divorce, or the death of a loved one.

Clinical psychologists use personal interviews, and they may also use diagnostic tests including blood tests and psychological tests. They may provide individual, family, or group therapy, or develop individual behavior-modification programs. Many specialize in working with people who have specific problems, such as post-traumatic stress or addiction. Psychologists may be less likely than marriage and family therapists or pastoral counselors to integrate spiritual issues into therapy. They do not typically prescribe medications, but often recommend medications that can be prescribed by a physician.

Pastoral Counselors

Although many women who attend religious services are aware that clergy typically have advanced religious training, many do not realize that religious training includes a significant amount of training in counseling and therapy. In addition, many clergy have advanced degrees in psychology and counseling. Pastoral counseling is a unique form of psychotherapy that uses spiritual resources as well as psychological understanding for healing and growth. Pastoral counselors are certified mental health professionals who also have had in-depth religious training.

The American Association of Pastoral Counselors (AAPC) sets standards for thousands of professionals in North America and around the world. The AAPC was founded in 1963 to certify pastoral counselors, accredit pastoral counseling centers, and approve training programs (see <www.aapc.org/about>). The organization is nonsectarian and respects the spiritual commitments and religious traditions of those who seek assistance without imposing counselor beliefs onto the clients. Women who would like counseling that integrates a spiritual perspective may prefer to seek help from a pastoral counselor.

THERAPY IN GROUPS

Even though millions of women are going through menopause, many feel alone and confused. They want to know that what they are experiencing is common for women their age and that it will not last forever.

I'm fifty-four and have been going through menopause since I was forty-six. The hot flashes were awful at first, but now seem to be getting better. But they're still with me! I never really understood what this phase means and what it does to your body. Even after almost nine years at this, I don't understand it all. After reading about menopause, I know now why I have all these tingling sensations, anxiety, loss of sex drive, the whole package. Now knowing that all this is quite normal has eased my mind and made me feel more "normal."

Similar to those who attend self-help groups or addiction recovery groups such as Alcoholics Anonymous, menopausal women can benefit from the experiences of others. Some local communities have support groups for women experiencing menopause. Women's groups, hospitals, and private clinics often offer information sessions, and there are numerous chat rooms and Internet discussion groups that use the online support group format to deal with issues faced by women during menopause.

"Girls Night Out": Female Bonding

Seeking out the experiences and opinions of friends and family can be extremely helpful. In today's society women often face personal conflict and guilt when it comes to meeting the demands of being a mother, spouse, employee, and a woman. Women may feel that their own concerns and health are a last priority when trying to fulfill everyone else's expectations and needs. As difficult as it may be to find the time, pampering herself or spending a "girls night out" can be one of the most rejuvenating gifts a woman can give herself. It can boost self-esteem, self-confidence, and energy. Talking about concerns and knowing that other women have similar feelings can be extremely reassuring. However, sometimes the nature of a group may change, becoming more of a hindrance than a help. Sessions might become complaining or blaming sessions rather than positive and encouraging. Ask yourself this: Do you come home from girls night out more angry and upset than relaxed and encouraged? If the answer is yes, it might be time to find a more supportive group.

OTHER CHOICES

Formal counseling and spending time with others can provide guidance and reassurance for women facing the changes of menopause. Some women may also seek out other ways of meeting personal needs during the menopausal transition, such as practicing yoga, meditation, and having massage therapy. Up to 30 percent of women use some form of complementary or alternative medicine to deal with health issues. Some studies show mild decreases in anxiety and depression symptoms in menopausal women using massage therapy or yoga exercises. Even more women report overall improvement in their sense of well-being when they use some or all of these therapies.

Menopause adds much (sometimes too much!) unpredictability to a woman's life. Many feel ill prepared to deal with these changes alone. To find hope and meaning and make sense of it all, a woman needs accurate information, support, and encouragement to enable her to find personal solutions to deal with this major life change. Finding a compatible counselor can help sort out all that is going on during these years. Ultimately, this will pay off in improved self-esteem, autonomy, and self-confidence—certainly good qualities to have in any developmental stage of life.

Chapter 5

Exercise: Moving Along the Menopause Journey

INTRODUCTION

As woman approach menopause they are likely to listen with a new sense of immediacy to recommendations about healthy lifestyles and the importance of exercise in promoting long-term health. During perimenopause the body reminds women—with hot flashes and night sweats—that the middle phase of life is ending and the next phase, ready or not, is beginning.

The immediate benefit of exercising is that it relieves many of the symptoms of perimenopause. Women who exercise have fewer or less severe hot flashes, more restful sleep, and less depression. One of the many changes taking place during the years leading to menopause is a decrease in circulating beta-endorphins. Even moderate physical exercise increases endorphins, improving a woman's overall sense of well-being. The long-term benefit is that exercise substantially decreases the risk of developing health problems that, for many of us, first become noticeable in our forties and fifties.

Moderate regular exercise can lower the risk for heart disease, adult-onset diabetes, and colon cancer. Simple strength training exercises can increase muscle strength and bone density to counter the effects of osteoarthritis and osteoporosis, and help the body use fat more efficiently. Stretching exercises, such as in yoga or warm-up and cool-down exercises, help ease joint pain and stiff-· ness and improve balance.

Bone loss leading to osteoporosis is one of the major health issues of women. Women begin losing bone density even before menopause, but loss accelerates after menopause for a number of reasons. Estrogen deficiency, inadequate calcium intake, and a decrease in physical activity all contribute. Exercise does not cure osteoporosis, but it can help in two ways: walking or other weight-bearing exercise slows bone loss and helps increase balance. Feeling stronger and having better balance makes one feel more secure. Fear of falling prevents many women from doing any kind of physical activity, and thus has broad implications for poor overall health. Sometimes it takes being diagnosed with low bone density to motivate women to exercise or take calcium. Women are far better off increasing physical activity (and taking extra calcium) sooner than later.

Regular moderate exercise can also help manage weight. The body uses fats much more efficiently if it is fit. If you are overweight, exercise can lower your risk for chronic illness or early death. If you are not overweight, you still need to be physically active. Controlling weight gain is just one of many benefits of exercise.

Exercise also helps reduce the negative effects of stress, which can make menopausal symptoms worse. Negative stress also increases blood pressure and strain on the heart, increases depressive mood, and lowers immune system function. A depressed immune system makes one more susceptible to both immediate and long-term health problems. Exercise helps restore physical and emotional balance.

At one time it was thought that the increase in health risk for women at midlife was caused mostly by hormonal changes. Now we know that much of the health risk is linked more to weight gain, particularly the gain in abdominal fat, which increases cardiovascular, metabolic, and cancer risks in both sexes, and to the decrease in physical activity linked to growing older. Over time the challenge to get back to the weight of our more active youth becomes more daunting. Despite all the media attention given to jogging or the lure of working out in stylish aerobics outfits, most women do not get the recommended amount of exercise to maintain a healthy lifestyle, much less to lose weight.

A steady transition from a sedentary lifestyle to structured vigorous activity, then to the stage of maintaining that level of activity, may be possible for some people. However, our own or family illness or other schedule-busting crises ("But I have to have it for school tomorrow!") may prevent a woman from keeping to her exercise schedule. Some women are determined to have their workout; they know when it works best for them, such as morning or evening, and will schedule their social or work life around those protected times. These women have developed a healthy sense of their own well-being. They may also live alone or in relatively independent relationships so they can protect that time, free of the misplaced feeling of guilt that they may be neglecting someone else's needs. More power to them.

Many women, however, are subject to, or subject themselves to, being "on call" for family, friends, or co-workers and deadlines, and have not yet learned that they can include their own health in the equation. Many women have not yet learned that their relationship with themselves is just *as important as* the relationships with other people or obligations. Therefore, it is not just permissible, but vital to add taking care of ourselves to the list of *things I must do.* One of the many qualities of women in younger generations is that they know their needs are important, too. The preceding generations helped them gain that insight, directly or indirectly. Now we can follow their lead in recognizing the need to distinguish between responsibility—the things we *must* do, and choice—the things we *can* do. We are responsible for improving our own health, and we can choose to do something about it.

About only 15 percent of women entering perimenopause participate in regular, vigorous workouts. This chapter is more for the millions of women at midlife who are still not comfortable with taking time for themselves until everybody else has been taken care of. Many women need extra encouragement to get started with exercise even though they know the benefits.

If we know exercise is good for our heart and bones, that it decreases the risk for other chronic diseases, and that it makes us feel better during menopause, why don't we "just do it," as the ads demand of us? Because many things must happen between *knowing* something is good for us and actually *doing* it. Any time we want to change our behavior—even when it means giving up something we know is not good for us, such as smoking, for the sake of something better, namely regular physical activity, we have to go through several stages of change.

STAGES OF CHANGE

Behavioral scientists have identified five stages of change: (1) precontemplation, (2) contemplation, (3) preparing for action, (4) taking action, and (5) maintaining the change. Moving from precontemplation to maintaining a change in behavior is rarely an uninterrupted progression. Most will slip back to a previous stage before they are ready to move into the next one. Knowing how change occurs can help keep one from getting stuck in the earliest stages, thinking he or she may not be capable of moving forward.

Small steps toward change can improve health and motivation. For example, just moving from the precontemplation stage to the preparation stage can improve blood pressure, total cholesterol, and a sense of well-being. If you are aware of the problems associated with lack of activity and are making even small changes, you are likely to have a more positive health profile than someone who is not thinking about it or is just beginning to think about it.

During perimenopause the processes involved in moving from sedentary behavior to maintaining regular physical activity seem more complex in the contemplation stage. As women come to terms with the transitions occurring at midlife, with all their emotional, physical, and spiritual implications, they can use the insight gained from reflection to further their resolve to set and accomplish healthy goals.

Precontemplation

My early perimenopausal symptoms are not that bad. I think I can deal with them. I've been relatively healthy until now, and I finally have a break from all the running around on behalf of children. Work and professional activities seem in better perspective. If there is one thing the passage of time has taught me, it is that work is only one part of my life. Until now I haven't really had time or been forced to think about my own long-term health or felt the urgency to restore balance in my daily life.

Stages of change for exercise are related to a number of perceptions and attitudes, including perceived social pressure, intention, attitudes, decisional balance (weighing pros and cons), and recognizing the harmful consequences of inactivity. So, what keeps us from getting enough exercise? Most of us believe we do not have time or enough social support. After all, who would take the children to ball practice or dance class if we don't do it? Other reasons may be bad weather that keeps us from taking a walk, or a schedule that is already overloaded, or too many family obligations. Yet good health relies on being physically active, so we need to become creative in figuring out how we can include it in our lives.

Contemplation

I'm having irregular periods, hot flashes, and night sweats. When I ask, "Is it hot in here, or is it just me?" a chorus of family members or co-workers respond, "It's just you!" My physician tells me it could be perimenopause. She reminds me that I need to be sure to eat a low-fat diet with at least five servings of fruits and vegetables a day. She also tells me I need to get more exercise, that I could stand to lose some weight, and tells me some of the health reasons that are so important. I have heard this litany before, but this time I listened more attentively. I think of all the reasons why exercising might be a problem, but now I'm also beginning to think about how I could overcome some of those barriers.

Stages of change for exercise can be related to self-perceived quality of life. The areas most strongly associated with perceptions of quality of life are physical functioning, general health perceptions, and vitality. Women who are least prepared to adopt regular exercise report the lowest levels of quality of life. Vitality and mental health are related to being active. Although intentions alone do not make us feel better about our lives, without them we are unlikely to take the next step. As we think through the positive and negative aspects of taking charge of our health, we begin to internalize more of the positive. We find that many of the barriers are of our own making, and, therefore, we can overcome them.

Preparing for Action

I know I should start an exercise program, but I just don't have time. Even if I could afford to join a health club, I'm not sleeping well and I feel too tired to go often enough to get my money's worth. I don't feel fit enough to start a vigorous exercise program. I know I need to get moving, but I want to do something that will help me feel better now. I just need to figure out how I can get started. Maybe if my son could switch his piano lesson to Wednesdays, I could start walking with my friend Lynn on Tuesdays and Thursdays.

The primary reason for inactivity among adults is lack of time. The most frequently cited cue to activity (what determines whether someone is active) is dissatisfaction with one's weight or appearance. Poor body image can be a catalyst to exercise, but if you feel embarrassed about the way you look you might also avoid exercising, at least in public. Just keep in mind that if you adopt a routine of moderate physical activity, you will be improving your health. If you feel healthy, you may be less likely to be as concerned about body image. Then you will be more likely to continue, and even increase, your level of activity. As for thinking there is no time in your life for exercise, consider this: The National Center for Chronic Disease Prevention and Health Promotion notes that people can benefit from participating in moderate-intensity activities only five times per week <www.cdc.gov/needphp/dnpa/physical/recommendations/index.htm>.

Besides the perception that there is not time for exercise, the Center also lists other common barriers to being physically active, and suggests some practical ways to overcome them (see Table 5.1).

Taking Action

Despite public health recommendations and media attention to the risks associated with being overweight, the majority of U.S. adults remain either overweight or obese. This is now recognized as a major public health crisis. After numerous studies that showed positive effects of moderate physical activity, recommendations have shifted from vigorous workouts to moderate levels of activity that could be incorporated into daily lifestyles. Studies of

TABLE 5.1. Barriers to being physically active.

Barriers	Suggestions for overcoming barriers
Lack of time	Look at your calendar or list all you do in one week. Find at least three, thirty-minute slots you can use for exercise. Begin by using that time to do some simple stretches, park farther from work or stores, or walk the dog.
Lack of support	Talk to your family and friends. They may want to join you as you start walking. Join a group of other women who may be starting to become more physically active and would walk with you. Carpool for children's activities so you can have a block of time.
Too tired	Think about the time of day you have the most energy. It may be before anyone else gets up. A brisk walk at lunch time will give you an energy boost for the afternoon. Do stretching exercises or yoga to refresh your body, mind, and spirit.
Bad weather	Think about balancing indoor and outdoor activities so you have options. Walk in a mall or gym or exercise at home.
Lack of resources	Find out about free or low-cost community resources such as exercise programs, tennis leagues, or walking trails. Stairs at home or work can be your stair machine.
Family obligations	Speak up about sharing household or caregiving responsibilities. Maybe no one else knows you need time for yourself. Learn to say no without feeling you have to apologize.

Source: Adapted from the recommendations for physical activity of The National Center for Chronic Disease Prevention and Health Promotion, 1999 <www.cdc.gov/needphp/dnpa/physical/life/overcome.htm>.

adults who had been sedentary but were otherwise healthy showed that moderate physical activity associated with lifestyle was as beneficial as a structured exercise program in improving physical activity, cardiorespiratory fitness, and blood pressure. That is good news for those who, whether for financial or social preferences, are less likely to join a gym or health club for intense workouts.

Maintaining Regular Physical Activity

One way to increase one's daily participation in exercise activity is to partake in lifestyle physical activity. The idea of "lifestyle physical activity" extends beyond leisure activities to include the accumulation of all leisure, occupational, and household activities of at least moderate physical intensity that are part of everyday life. Such activities can be planned or unplanned. It is reassuring to know one does not have to do long-distance running or extreme sports to get and stay fit. Of course that is good news for older Americans, especially for those approaching or beyond menopause. Current recommendations greatly expand our exercise options.

Now that we know that regular moderate activity can, in the long run, be just as beneficial, we can begin to see the possibility of setting goals for physical activity that can fit into our lives. We may even be better able to maintain a more moderate level of activity than some who throw themselves into a rigorous exercise regimen only to give up after a few weeks or months because of injury or an unexpected disruption of an exercise schedule. Regular, conscious lifestyle activities, such as going for a brisk walk after dinner or lunch, doing housework or yard work, or taking the stairs instead of the elevator can add up to the recommended thirty minutes a day.

The Centers for Disease Control and Prevention has classified levels of activity (amount of energy expended) into general categories that include daily activities (see Tables 5.2 and 5.3).

For many of us, barriers to recreational exercise include taking care of family members, feeling too tired, not having time, and not

TABLE 5.2. Recreational activity or exercise.

Activity	Light	Moderate	Vigorous
Walking	Slowly in the house or yard, shopping	Briskly, downstairs or down a hill	Racewalking, jogging or running, hiking
Bicycling	Less than 5 mph on level terrain, stationary bike with light effort	5 to 10 mph, level terrain or few hills, stationary bike with moderate effort	More than 10 mph, lots of hills
Dancing	Stretching and slow warm-up, slow ballroom dancing	Fast ballroom dancing, line dancing, tap dancing	Square dancing, aerobic dance class
Tennis, table tennis	Warm-up before a match, leisure game of table tennis	Tennis doubles, competitive table tennis	Tennis singles
Golf	Riding a golf cart, driving range, miniature golf	Carrying clubs or wheeling a golf bag	
Swimming	Floating, treading water slowly	Swimming, diving, water-skiing, snorkeling, surfing	Laps, water jogging, treading water rapidly, scuba diving
Skiing or skating		Downhill with light effort, ice skating at a leisurely pace, snowmobiling	Racing downhill, speedskating, sledding

having a safe place to exercise. Other barriers may be financial. However, in the spectrum of options, health clubs are not the only place we can exercise, especially when we think of it in terms of physical activity and not just leisure-time, organized classes. Less expensive alternatives include parks and recreation programs, exercise tapes or DVDs we can check out at the library or purchase for our own use, bicycling, and the least expensive form of physical activity—walking.

TABLE 5.3. General physical activity.

Activity	Light	Moderate	Vigorous
Housework	Dusting, vacuuming, sweeping, making beds, cooking or serving food, washing dishes, folding or putting away laundry	Scrubbing the floor or bathtub on hands and knees, sweeping outside, cleaning garage, washing windows, moving light furniture	Moving or pushing heavy furniture (75 lbs or more), carrying items 25 lbs or more upstairs
Gardening	Pruning, weeding, using a riding mower, weeding while sitting or kneeling	Raking, digging, planting trees, pushing a power lawn mower, stacking wood	Heavy shoveling, climbing and trimming trees, pushing a nonmotorized lawn mower
Playing with children	Sitting while playing; dressing, bathing, or feeding a child	Walking, running, carrying a small child while walking, walking while pushing a child in a stroller, carrying a toddler upstairs	Running longer distances with a child, jogging while pushing a stroller, carrying a larger child upstairs
Occupation	General office work, sales, driving a car or light truck, assembly-line work, patient care	Home repair, driving a heavy truck or equipment, mail delivery on foot, waiting tables, packing, moving patients, physical therapy	Long periods of running, pushing or pulling heavy objects, strenuous total body effort, lifting or carrying heavy objects, teaching aerobics

MIND, BODY, AND SPIRIT

In combination with weight-bearing exercise to protect against osteoporosis and resistance exercises to increase muscle mass, flexibility exercises such as yoga can also help alleviate symptoms of menopause. Yoga can also help relieve stress. Stress keeps our focus on the external part of our lives and prevents us from being able to distinguish between events that are within our control and those that are not. Yoga and meditation can help maintain a positive attitude and sense of empowerment. We can then begin to make the most of this time in our lives to take stock and renew a commitment to our own well-being.

Yoga helps balance the endocrine system and improves strength and flexibility, which are essential to getting the most benefit from all other types of exercise. Certain yoga positions, such as headstands or shoulder stands, are particularly effective in lessening the severity of hot flashes and night sweats. Yoga in the evening can help you let go of the problems of the day. When you are relaxed, consciously monitoring your breathing, meditating, or prayerful, you are more likely to be able to focus on the positive aspects of your life and cope with the negative. The key to finding hope beyond current circumstances is balance—physical, emotional, and spiritual.

Chapter 6

Menopause and the Workplace

Experiencing menopausal symptoms at work can be doubly stressful, with daily job pressures complicating the challenge of waiting out a hot flash or momentary loss of concentration. At home, families are expected to care about how mother, wife, or grandmother feels, but what happens outside the protected family setting? At home women may be able to find a quiet place when they need to deal with a sudden burst of emotion. Work, on the other hand, is almost always a public activity. Given that as a society we are still battling stereotypes associated with raging hormones and aging women, it is not surprising that women may hesitate to talk openly about menopause in the workplace. Many women fear that expressing a potential need for special accommodation for fluctuating hormones might be regarded as further rationalization for marginalizing women.

CHANGES IN THE WORKPLACE

About 65 percent of all American women are employed, and that percentage is increasing. Each year since 2000 about 2 million women have entered the menopausal transition. This adds up to a large number of hot flashes or other menopausal symptoms on the job; a formidable issue that needs to be addressed in the American business world.

Many changes have taken place in the workplace. The increase in the number of on-site day care facilities, flexible work schedules, and telecommuting are some examples. Many businesses have found that these changes in the way people work can be good for both morale and the bottom line. Corporations now also invest millions of dollars per year on seminars and workshops on diversity, gender issues, communication, time management, stress management, and team building. In the past these may have been considered the "softer" issues of employee relations and development.

Menopause Gaining Attention

Many businesses and corporations (e.g., Daimler Chrysler Corporation) include menopause among topics presented in wellness programs in the workplace. Workshops for businesswomen, human resources managers, and CEOs about menopause in the workplace are available. Manufacturers of hormone replacement drugs and herbal remedies for menopausal symptoms cosponsor some of the meetings and thus have a stake in managing menopause. Some of the consultants on menopause in the workplace are women whose own negative experiences motivated them to enter this new field. They have a vast and receptive audience among the growing number of menopausal baby boomers and from some employers concerned with the cost benefits of dealing with this broader definition of wellness.

One indication of the changing climate in major corporations are the several articles on menopause-related topics published over the past few years by *Fortune* magazine, one of the leading magazines on business. That may have something to do with the increasing number of women entering the workforce, as well as the influence of greater numbers of women in top positions. Both women and men have done much to change corporate culture in the past few decades, but old habits and stereotypes die hard both in and outside the boardroom. Beyond the workplace, discussions among women of the menopause experience are becoming more common. In 1991, when Gail Sheehy first published her landmark book on menopause, *The Silent Passage* (most recently revised in 1998), the topic was still taboo in public or mixed company. Even now, the experiences of other women—not necessarily the medical community—are the main sources for information about menopause. Women have formed support groups among friends and through discussions over the Internet. Many Web sites based in the United States and Europe are devoted to the subject. However, talking about the fears and frustrations of menopausal symptoms outside such supportive groups is not so easy.

Consultants who specialize in dealing with menopause at work—a major indication of the changing culture in corporations—suggest confiding in a supervisor or co-workers about what you are going through. That may be difficult for many reasons, including lack of confidentiality in the workplace and fear of being considered incapable of handling the job. Some women tell of crying for "no reason," being drenched with perspiration during meetings, or feeling tired and disoriented during the day because of poor sleep the previous night. They may worry that menopause will make them seem less capable of doing their work and thus hurt the careers they have spent years building.

MANAGING MENOPAUSE AT WORK

In the United States, a leading organization for working women (Business and Professional Women/USA) developed a program to help companies work with their female employees to manage menopause at work. A major emphasis of the program was to educate both male and female employees about menopause to help dispel some of the myths and stereotypes. It also advocates for health insurance companies to cover the range of treatment options for menopausal symptoms. One of the organization's most important messages for women and their employers was that symptoms are temporary. Most accommodations, if any are needed at all, are relatively simple and inexpensive. They include providing small fans or comfortable temperatures in work areas, cool water, and bathroom breaks as needed.

The National Institute on Aging has suggested a number of ways to help manage menopausal symptoms at work. The following list is adapted from the National Institute of Aging's "Menopause" <www.niapublications.org>:

- Sip ice water at the beginning of a hot flash.
- Use a cool damp cloth for hands, forehead, or neck.
- Wear layered clothing and remove layers when a hot flash starts.
- Wear cotton clothes (they release heat and absorb moisture).
- Cut down on hot beverages and spicy foods.
- Keep *one* "to-do" list by your telephone as a reminder of commitments you have made but may be afraid of forgetting.
- Use deep-breathing exercises to reduce stress and to refocus (especially before a meeting or presentation).
- Try to keep moving during the day to reduce fatigue from sitting too long.
- Cut down on salt and caffeine.

Self-confidence tends to falter during menopausal symptoms. To counter self-doubt, make a list of accomplishments and keep it in a daily calendar, desk drawer, or inside a locker. During stress at work it may be difficult to remember positive experiences and call on those successes to get through a rough patch during the workday.

Several methods of relieving stress are particularly useful in dealing with menopausal symptoms at work. It takes only a few minutes to do simple stretching exercises such as resting your chin on your chest to gently stretch the neck and rolling the shoulders forward and backward slowly to relax your arms and upper back. During the same few minutes, practice conscious breathing—inhale deeply through the nose for a few seconds, then exhale slowly through the mouth. The combination of exercise and conscious breathing should help relieve muscle tightness and improve concentration and focus.

Focus may seem impossible when menopausal symptoms, along with the unrelenting stresses of work, feel so overwhelming. With practice, focusing techniques can help the process of sorting out the causes of anxiety or frustration, both of which can trigger sudden bursts of anger or tears during "menopause moments" at work or at home.

Relieving Stress

One method of managing stress is to use a relaxation response when the body signals an overload such as a rapid heartbeat, tight shoulder muscles, or a feeling of panic. The relaxation response, as recommended by Herbert Benson, president of the Mind/Body Medical Institute in Massachusetts, begins with repeating a word, a short phrase, or a prayer to break the cycle of racing, nonproductive thoughts (Benson and Klipper, 1975). When the mind is calmer, it is possible to focus on breathing evenly to ease tension in the neck and shoulders. As the feeling of panic begins to subside, think about whether the situation warrants the anger. In a typical office situation, for example, many co-workers and managers may be requesting immediate results on a project. In an effort to please everyone, a woman may say, "Yes, I can help with that" so many times that the volume of work and deadlines create an avalanche of unfinished paperwork. Is the direction of anger outward, at co-workers, or inward, because it is hard to say no or to ask for help in setting priorities and completing multiple tasks? As a woman enters the menopausal years she may be starting to feel frustrated by what she perceives as having to be available for everyone just because they ask. Think about the person who might say, "Yes, I can probably work that in *next week*," or, depending on who is doing the asking, "I will not be able to help because of so many prior commitments." Some people may ask for the impossible, but few actually expect to get it—particularly when they know the situation. The woman who says, "Yes, but not now" or "That won't be possible given your deadline" is likely to be both respected and vilified. She may also be healthier and better able to manage menopausal symptoms on the job. Many women contribute to their own impossible situations by thinking they can work miracles with space and time. A woman can still "have it all" and "do it all." Just not all at once. That principle applies equally at home and at work.

Coping with Anxiety and Frustration

As evident in so much of what has been written about menopause, anxiety and frustration can be traced more to life events during midlife than to female hormones. Setting aside time to reflect on just one aspect of life, such as work, is a good start for calming an anxious mind. It is also good practice for learning to reflect (not worry incessantly) about the much more complex relationships among family or friends.

You can begin by just making a few notes about how you felt during an unsettling situation at work. It could be a co-worker making a joke about aging women or thermostat wars in the office (for the hundredth time!), or when your willingness to help finish someone else's project keeps you at the office while they go home on time because they have a family commitment (again!). Write about these issues for brief periods without getting stuck in analyzing your feelings. That will come later. Writing down your feelings first helps you step outside the situation so you can think about it more objectively, and then you will be more able to find an appropriate way to address the situation with the other people involved to try to keep it from happening again. Sometimes we worry a problem into a monumental issue when a word about how we felt and why could quickly solve the problem.

For example, sometimes we laugh about menopausal moments. When someone else picks up the routine and uses it numerous times, it begins to feel as if it were an assault. Women may fret about what co-workers will think if they decide, in their "menopausal assertive way," that they don't want to go along with the joke or the extra work. Women may think others need to know the effect of what they say. People at work may not be aware of fallout from their behavior, even if they are in one of the companies that have wellness seminars on menopause. Talking about the situation when you can approach the subject calmly can make you feel better and, at the same time, help relieve some of the stress of dealing with menopausal symptoms at work. Self-understanding will grow with practice in expressing feelings. Women who find it too difficult to break the worry cycle and self-doubt would likely benefit from working with one of the counselors described in Chapter 4. A trained counselor can guide the search for self-understanding. Only with self-understanding is perspective possible, paving the way toward peace and balance, even at work. The process may be painful, but it can have far-reaching and perhaps unexpectedly positive results.

FINDING FULFILLMENT

Questions are bound to arise in dealing with menopausal symptoms at work, such as, How much of the stress do I want to manage? What if I no longer want to put so much energy into coping with stress at my job? How can I find out what I really want to do? It might be working in a different job. It could also mean finding fulfillment and deep satisfaction in nurturing another part of your life, and balancing the meaning of work in a broader context.

Katherine Ramsland, in her book *Bliss: Writing to Find Your True Self* (2000), has written a useful guide to self-discovery. She defines bliss as becoming fully engaged with your life. The goal is to achieve emotional, spiritual, and psychological balance. She advises that to discover bliss, you have to begin by finding out what is important to you, what your values are, and what you want from your life. The process entails reflecting on different experiences, including the times you felt stuck in your life or work and the times you felt good about something you did. Then you can reflect on the differences in your feelings in both situations and how those feelings affected other parts of your life. Insight gained from reflecting on experiences opens up possibilities for dealing with similar situations in the future. The goal, of course, is to work toward more experiences that evoke good feelings. Gaining self-knowledge requires commitment and patience, working through the process step by step.

A final note on work and the "change of life" is that there is hope in knowing that many others, both men and women, are struggling with the physical and emotional effects of midlife. So far, women have an advantage because they have more information about midlife passages. They can gain comfort in learning about the process taking place in the transition to menopause. Only recently has research on male midlife issues indicated similar symptoms among men, including decreasing hormone levels, fatigue, weight gain, short-term memory loss, irritability, indecisiveness, depression, lowering of sexual desire, and fears of sexual potency loss. Both men and women may feel a kind of undefined restlessness, a longing for "something else." For better or worse, we are not alone.

Chapter 7

Spiritual Issues Facing
Women at Midlife

Why focus on the spiritual issues of life at menopause and at midlife? First, many women are religious and likely to regard spirituality as an important part of their daily lives. Furthermore, the challenges of menopause and the midlife bring a new perspective and a new energy to the search for hope and meaning. Dr. Christiane Northrup has pointed out that menopause is an opportunity for spiritual growth in her book *The Wisdom of Menopause* (2001).

> In some cultures, such as that of Hindu India, midlife is a time associated with the serious pursuit of the spiritual dimensions of life. I see something comparable occurring in this country, where the vast majority of attendees at conferences on the connection between the body and soul are midlife women. With our child rearing years behind us, our creative energies are freed. Our search for life's meaning begins to take on new urgency, and we begin to experience ourselves as potential vessels of the Spirit. (p. 71)

Midlife is sometimes a struggle—but does it have to be? Is the hopeless feeling that so many women have inevitable? The answer, and a big part of the motivation for the writing of this book, is no. Many women often face the challenges of midlife without the help of spiritual comfort and support. Walt Larimore (2003), a noted author and physician, has said that neglecting the spiritual side of your personal life is similar to driving a car that has one flat tire. This chapter discusses women's spiritual dimensions and how they can learn to activate their spiritual resources. The chapter will review the most common spiritual issues of midlife and review recent research regarding the role of spirituality in anxiety, depression, and physical illness. How health care providers can approach spiritual issues in a sensitive way, and how you can work with your doctor in gaining access to the spiritual resources that are available will also be addressed.

FINDING SPIRITUAL RESOURCES

Women often suffer through the stages of menopause without making use of spiritual help. For example, women come to our offices with physical complaints of headaches, abdominal pain, or hot flashes, without realizing that their underlying problem is spiritual—it is emotional pain that has rocked them to their core and made them question life's meaning. What makes the situation worse is that they do not realize that their problems must be addressed from the spiritual as well as the physical side. They have tried unsuccessfully to create more energy and reduce emotional pain and stress on their own. Such women are strong, self-reliant, and have often borne the brunt of family responsibilities for many years. They are not used to asking for help.

When we ask them how they are coping with midlife's many challenges, they respond, "I just try to handle it." When we ask them to elaborate they often have trouble explaining what "just handle it" means. We get the sense that it means that they internalize stress and call on the last of their emotional and physical reserves to cope. When they arrive in the office their reserve tank is empty. "Handling it" is one way to cope, but there are more effective methods.

Jamie's Story

Jamie was forty-nine years old and starting to have some hot flashes. Her periods were irregular, but the symptoms were not intolerable. She came to my office mainly for a blood pressure checkup. Her blood pressure was high (160/98), which was unusual for her.

Her blood pressure was usually in the 135/85 range, and she was good about coming in for checkups. I asked her, "How are things? What's been going on?" and tears formed in the corner of one eye. Then she told me her story.

Her son had been a drug dealer and user, and was put in jail. She did not complain that he had been incarcerated; in fact, she said it was a chance for him to "get straightened out." She was very excited that he would be getting out soon, after being in prison for three years. She and her sister found a little apartment for him and went to many garage sales to find furnishings. They could not afford many new things. She spent what little savings she had to get a brand new couch and a small stereo. After all of her shopping, she was very proud of how the place looked. Furthermore, she knew how important it was for him to not fall in with the wrong people when he got out. He needed to stay busy and productive. So she talked to a friend and found her son a job at a factory right across the street from the new apartment. He would be able to walk to work.

After her son had been out of jail a week she got a call from her friend at the factory. Did she know where her son was? He had not been to work for three days. Jamie picked up her sister, and they went to the apartment immediately. The couch and the stereo were gone, the curtains were gone, and every room was stripped of any articles that could be sold. Her son had sold all of it for drugs. He was back on the streets. Jamie sobbed uncontrollably. In her eyes was the question, "Where do I turn?"

I took her hand and tried to console her. I knew that the answer for her would not be found in blood pressure pills or a prescription for the latest designer hormone, although some of those things might have been medically indicated. Her problem is best understood in a spiritual context rather than a medical one. Her struggle for answers would involve addressing spiritual questions as much as emotional, psychological, and medical ones. Only by taking time to consider life's ultimate meaning would she be able to put her recent life events in a healing context. Physicians cannot provide those answers for patients, but they can prompt them to seek spiritual answers. I asked Jamie, "Where have you turned for hope, for strength?" Her sobbing calmed for a moment, and she looked up and said, "To the Lord."

Our conversation continued, and she shared that she had religion-based spiritual resources to draw upon. Despite her emotional tears in my office she was holding up remarkably well. She was involved in a Christian church congregation, was getting meals delivered to her home by church members, and was receiving family support as well. She was receiving both social and spiritual support from her friends.

Many women are not so fortunate to be connected to such a supportive network. She did get her prescription for her blood pressure medicine refilled that day, and promised to do a better job of taking it regularly.

Many of you can sympathize with Jamie, perhaps not with the details of her situation, but with pouring yourself out for someone and then feeling betrayed. The stress of daily life with teenagers, husbands who don't help around the house, grandma's illness, crazy hormone fluctuations, and a demanding boss at work conspire to rob you of all energy. Of course you have headaches, ulcers, hot flashes, and backaches! When was the last time you slept eight hours? When was the last time you took a long hot bath? When was the last time you went outside and walked (or jogged) for forty-five minutes? When was the last time you meditated or prayed?

We know you want the bath, the long walk, and the sleep, but how many of you realize you need to take the time for prayer or meditation? To ponder life and its meaning? To focus on your spiritual side? To consider whether there is a force out there (or in you) that is greater than you? Jamie took the time and was reaping a spiritual and emotional benefit.

Women do not look toward spiritual resources during menopause for several reasons. One is that many women like to rely on their own inner strength. It has worked well for many years—or has it? Women make twice as many visits to the doctor as men, take more medicine, and have higher rates of depression than men. Perhaps "handling it" is not working as well as women think. Many women could benefit from recognizing that what they are doing is not working. A new level of spiritual attention can do wonders for the soul.

Another reason some women do not turn to the spiritual is that they do not believe it will help. This feeling of futility is not exclusive to any particular religious tradition or spiritual approach. Many spiritually centered women serve others and pour out their love for others in a way inspired by their faith tradition. However, many of these same women do not believe that their God is interested in their personal spiritual needs. "Why would God be interested in me?" they ask. "God is concerned with wars and cancer and saving people in Africa, not me."

Jamie would say that this is a situation that requires you to have faith. Despite her grief about her son, she was able to share with me the basis for her belief that "things would work out for the best in the end. If God knows, as it says in the scriptures, about every hair on your head, every flower, every tree in the field, then I know he knows about me, too," Jamie shared. Whatever your faith or spiritual tradition, seeing life's ups and downs in the spiritual context is almost always uplifting and hope giving. The strongest and most resilient women in my practice are those that possess a strong spiritual faith.

Another reason many women do not seek spiritual support is because they are very focused on others. A lot of women spend most of their waking hours taking care of other people in their lives. They cook, clean, wash, attend ballet concerts and baseball games, and often maintain part-time or full-time jobs as well. Women are the servants and backbones of families. This is not recognized enough, celebrated enough, or appreciated enough. This unselfishness is a marvelous and noble trait. Doctors and therapists are reluctant to confront or criticize women regarding this trait in any way. However, there is a high price for this total outward focus—many women pay less attention to their own health and particularly their own spiritual needs. In general, women need to attend to *themselves,* as well as to others, so that they can maintain their own health and perspective.

Finally, it is important to realize that spirituality is distinctive. The strength that comes from personal religious and spiritual beliefs is unique. It is more than social support from religious or supportive friends; the hope and strength of spirituality is there when the friends are not. The sacred provides hope long after secular hope is gone. Religious and spiritual beliefs provide explanations for events and new perspectives that cannot be provided by nonreligious or nonspiritual systems. Rediscover your spiritual and religious roots for their own sake, and realize that the health and well-being they provide are added benefits of the peace that is their main objective.

Charlene's Story

Charlene was diagnosed with diabetes when she was thirty years old. For ten years she struggled with the disease, and mostly fought a losing battle. Her weight was on a constant up and down cycle and her blood sugar was never well controlled. She never seemed to find the time to exercise. She and her husband were not getting along well. When she had her daughter she thought that event would bring them closer together. However, it did not. Her husband left her and she began to feel very alone. She looked many places for inspiration, and she says she had no dramatic conversion. There were no visions, no angels, and no bright lights from the sky. Nevertheless, when she began to focus on the spiritual upbringing and faith of her youth, her life began to turn around. I met her in the office when one of the residents in the training program in which I teach asked me to meet her. The resident was very impressed by her excellent diabetes control and her positive attitude. When I met her she was glowing. She told me about her new lease on life and her forty-five-pound weight loss, which she had kept off for two years. She and her daughter were doing well despite the earlier hardships.

Charlene volunteered to assist our medical practice with a twelve-week class for other women with diabetes, and was an inspiration to everyone. Her enthusiasm and energy were infectious and her smile was permanent, no matter what was happening in her life on a given day. She constantly reminded the others in the group to keep a long-term spiritual perspective, to focus on the positive, and to take the time to keep themselves healthy.

One of the best ways to convince women that they need rest, self-attention, and spiritual renewal is to talk to them about the need to care for themselves if they want to continue to care for others. Sometimes women are trying to be as unselfish in their personal spiritual lives as they are with their families. However, neglecting oneself completely leads to more feelings of stress and a greater risk of medical illness. Being attentive to spiritual issues such as meaning, priorities, and long-term perspective enables women to focus on the bigger picture and to value themselves enough to attend to their own health.

WHY ATTEND TO THE SPIRITUAL ASPECTS OF LIFE AT MENOPAUSE?

Does attentiveness to the spiritual and religious side of life have anything to offer to people who are not in crisis? Is religion only for people in trouble? Is there a link between positive emotions, health, and spirituality?

The answer to these questions, based on our clinical experience and recent research, is that attention to spiritual and religious issues is a boost for people who are doing well as well as for those who are in crisis. Michael McCullough, a psychologist and researcher at the University of Miami, has found a substantial connection between spirituality and positive emotions. People who are more spiritual are also more grateful, more humble, more hopeful, and more likely to be volunteers. Spirituality promotes peace, harmony, civility, and forgiveness. Dr. McCullough's groundbreaking work on forgiveness emphasizes the importance of forgiveness in everyday life. Highly spiritual people are more likely to practice forgiveness on a daily basis than less spiritual people, and thus are more likely to be emotionally healthy. It is not that spiritual people are pushovers who always let people take advantage of them, it is simply that they are more likely to move forward in their relationships without the baggage of unforgiveness weighing them down. Peace and not holding a grudge are valued more than correctness or revenge.

Try this exercise. Write down three things you are grateful for each day for two weeks. If you are similar to the people in Dr. McCullough's experiment you will feel better and more positive. Your own spirituality will grow, and you will have more peace within. It is fascinating to consider that an exercise as simple as writing down aspects of life for which you are thankful would have such a positive and profound effect, but it is true. Writing down three things for which you are thankful, a type of journaling, can have a similar beneficial effect as meditation for ten to twenty minutes a day. The results of research on daily meditation (Harmon and Myers, 1999) and gratitude journaling (Pennebaker and

Seagal, 1999) confirm that their benefits are very similar. Gratitude and forgiveness are good for your health!

SPIRITUALITY AND HEALTH: IS THERE A PHYSIOLOGICAL CONNECTION?

Evidence of a biochemical connection between spirituality, stress, and forgiveness has recently been found, and may provide more evidence of the positive benefits of spirituality even for people not experiencing a crisis. People who are more religious and spiritual have lower levels of cortisol, a stress hormone (Dedert et al., 2004). Such people also have lower rates of anxiety and depression. People who regularly practice forgiveness also have lower cortisol levels. Many researchers suspect that religiousness, spirituality, and forgiveness may be linked to mental and physical health through physiological pathways. Furthermore, people who are higher in spirituality/religiousness are also more able to deal with stressful situations. People who use their spirituality to help cope with stress have less "overreactive" cortisol levels, which means the levels are less prone to rise under stress (Ironson et al., 2002).

People who attend religious services have also been found to have lower levels of C-reactive protein, a protein in the blood stream associated with increased risk of heart attacks. In people at higher risk of heart attack, such as those with diabetes, the relationship of religion and C-reactive protein is even stronger (King, Mainous, Steyer, Pearson, 2001; King, Mainous, Pearson, 2002). Those who attend religious services once a week or more also have stronger immune systems. These biochemical connections were not investigated by researchers to "prove" the existence of God or a divine force in the world, but they were done to show that there are scientific links between religious and spiritual beliefs and practice and dealing with stress, links that should interest women who are facing a high-stress period of transition in their lives. Because many women at midlife are under increased stress from hormonal changes and life events, it may be comforting to know that there is scientific evidence for what many already know from experience—that attention to spirituality is associated with positive emotions, gratitude, hope, and ultimately better health.

HOW DO I BEGIN TO ADDRESS SPIRITUAL ISSUES?

How can women best get started with addressing spirituality? What we are about to suggest may be challenging. You are going to have to take some *time off.* We mean some mental time off. Schedule some personal thinking time, time for reflection. Dealing with spiritual issues will require some of your undivided attention. Consider the following issues, one at a time.

Forgiveness

This is essentially a spiritual issue. Forgiveness is not the same as paying a debt, but it is similar. Have you ever owed money to the bank? How did you feel when you paid it off? It felt good, didn't it? A real cause for celebration. You paid off your credit card—hoorah! Then consider this possibility: suppose the bank informed you that you did not owe the money anymore. Wow. That would feel good, too. Maybe even better than good, especially if you owed a lot. However, it might bring other emotions also. You might begin to ask, "Why did I deserve this?" and think "I feel guilty accepting this generous offer." You might even want to refer your friends to that bank out of gratitude. You see? It's more complicated than it first appears.

Dr. Francis MacNutt, a minister, healer, and noted author, states in his book *Healing* (1974, 1999), that forgiveness is the first and deepest kind of healing. His is a decidedly religious view:

> What I have come to see, though, is how intimately the for- ·
> giveness of sins is connected with bodily and emotional heal-
> ing. They are not separate . . . there is good evidence, then,
> that there is a very natural connection between much of our

sickness and our spiritual and emotional health. (pp. 169-171)

MacNutt is convinced that inner healing begins with forgiveness—forgiving others, and also forgiving oneself. Inner healing and spiritual healing begin with forgiveness. Forgive and be forgiven. You will feel a burden lifted, and then you will be able to begin a total body healing and restoration of balance. Take the personal meditation and prayer time you need to address this spiritual issue. It is the foundation for experiencing what MacNutt calls "salvation and healing at the deepest level" (p. 169).

Forgiveness is also the cornerstone of Alcoholics Anonymous (AA). The organization was started by people struggling with addiction to alcohol who discovered that they needed to explore "twelve steps" to get control of their lives again and away from the influence of addiction. The organization is a person-to-person movement. They have no building or national dues. You will find a local AA chapter in most phone books. An AA Web site is available which contains basic information (www.aa.org). It is a volunteer organization, and is focused on group meetings and working through the twelve steps toward healing (see Exhibit 7.1). When you read the twelve steps it is easy to see the focus on forgiveness. The process is one that started with AA and the struggle to be free from alcohol addiction, but the steps are now used by a variety of groups including Narcotics Anonymous and Overeaters Anonymous. The steps chart a path of self-discovery that would benefit many midlife women, even if they do not struggle with alcohol.

Grace

Grace is similar to forgiveness, but it goes further. Grace has a fragrance and attraction all its own. Grace means all the blame is gone. It means you are starting over with a clean slate. Forgiveness starts it, but grace takes it further. It is similar to having total amnesia for the bad part of a situation and remembering only the good part.

EXHIBIT 7.1. The Twelve Steps

1. We admitted we were powerless over alcohol—that our lives had become unmanageable.
2. Came to believe that a power greater than ourselves could restore us to sanity.
3. Made a decision to turn our will and our lives over to the care of God as we understood Him.
4. Made a searching and fearless moral inventory of ourselves.
5. Admitted to God, to ourselves, and to another human being the exact nature of our wrongs.
6. Were entirely ready to have God remove all these defects of character.
7. Humbly asked Him to remove our shortcomings.
8. Made a list of all persons we had harmed, and became willing to make amends to them all.
9. Made direct amends to such people wherever possible, except when to do so would injure them or others.
10. Continued to take personal inventory and when we were wrong, promptly admitted it.
11. Sought through prayer and meditation to improve our conscious contact with God as we understood Him, praying only for knowledge of His will for us and the power to carry that out.
12. Having had a spiritual awakening as the result of these steps, we tried to carry this message to alcoholics and to practice these principles in all our affairs.

The Twelve Steps are reprinted with permission of Alcoholics Anonymous World Services, Inc. (AAWS). Permission to reprint the Twelve Steps does not mean that AAWS has reviewed or approved the contents of this publication, or that AAWS necessarily agrees with the views expressed herein. AA is a program of recovery from alcoholism *only*—use of the Twelve Steps in connection with programs and activities which are patterned after AA, but which address other problems, or in any other non-AA context, does not imply otherwise.

Randy Alcorn expresses this idea well in his book *The Grace and Truth Paradox* (2003). He tells about an ancient Greek tradition of writing the word *teleo* across certificates of debt when they were cancelled. It meant *paid in full*. That is the thought behind grace, and it is refreshing for those struggling with guilt, past regrets, or current feelings of unforgiveness. Alcorn goes on to explain the story behind the beloved hymn "Amazing Grace." The

song is sung in many churches every week, with love and gratitude. However, many people may not know that John Newton, a
cruel slave ship captain who transported slaves to America, wrote
the song. The words of one of the verses may resonate with you
now:

> Thru many dangers, toils, and snares, I have already come;
> 'Tis grace that brought me safe thus far, and grace will lead
> me home.

Someone who turned his life around spiritually wrote those inspi-
rational words.

Spiritual Connectedness

Fortunately, you do not need to take the journey alone. Connecting with others is a natural and healthy part of dealing with the
spiritual issues that women face during menopause. Reconnecting
with your spiritual and religious roots may be a helpful way to deal
with the stress and challenges of menopause.

JG had two problems—menopause and a rebellious daughter. Between the two, she was not sure which was driving her crazier. Her
periods were starting to skip months, and she could not tolerate
estrogen-replacement medications. She knew she had mood swings
and could become upset more easily. On top of that situation, her
daughter was popular and had a lot of friends, not all of whom met
with her approval. Her daughter's staying out late at night brought
more anxiety for JG, amid worries of car accidents or worse. Who
was she with and what were they doing? Was her daughter safe?
When she came to see me it was for a pregnancy test for her daughter. When I told them it was positive, JG's head just sagged. After
dealing with the immediate issues regarding her daughter, JG returned to see me separately to talk about her anxiety. I found out that
her connections with other women were a big part of her coping style.
She met weekly with a women's group, and related that she derived a
lot of spiritual and emotional support from meeting and sharing with
others.

JG's story illustrates a common finding: reliance on and connecting with other people for emotional and spiritual support can greatly improve one's outlook. We mentioned previously in the chapter that attending religious services is associated with improved immune system function. In addition, research has found that people who connect with others actually *live longer.* This is true even after taking into account age, smoking, and other health habits. Social and spiritual support through sharing with others creates a strong positive influence for many midlife women (Oman and Reed, 1998; Hummer et al., 1999; Musick et al., 2004).

The previous statements in no way discount the importance of personal devotion and practice in the lives of women. Women who pray regularly and meditate feel better and are less likely to be depressed. Personal devotion to God recently has been found to exert a protective effect on psychological distress (Levin 2002). However, the spiritual support and connectedness associated with attending religious services has a benefit that is above and beyond these factors. Taking the spiritual journey alone is possible, but going on the journey with other like-minded people can be even more rewarding.

SPIRITUALITY FOR ITS OWN SAKE: THE PARADOX

We cannot leave this subject without a word of caution about spirituality for its own sake. There is a paradox in dealing with spirituality and health that puts doctors and therapists in an awkward position. Although there are several health benefits to being more attentive to the spiritual side of your life, *you will not see the rewards if you pursue spirituality only because of the health benefits.* You must pursue spirituality for its own sake. None of the benefits will accrue if you only go through the motions. Researchers explain the phenomenon by differentiating between two kinds of religious commitment, *extrinsic* and *intrinsic.* Extrinsic religiosity, for example, is going to church for the purpose of earthly benefits, social connections, or even better health. Intrinsic religious commitment is an internal, sincere desire to seek a connection with God and to seek spiritual answers to life's questions. The associations with better health described in this book are associated only with the intrinsic kind of spiritual/religious commitment. Your spiritual passage must be a sincere one that comes from the heart. We have no prescription or magic formula for you to follow. Doctors cannot prescribe religiousness to patients. We can only explain that the answers are beyond medication and that coping with the challenges of menopause is a spiritual and emotional expedition as well as a physical one. Faith and commitment must come from within.

SPIRITUALITY AND HEALTH CARE PROVIDERS

How to Relate to Health Care Providers
About Spiritual Issues

Many health care providers do not pay attention to the idea that some women have spiritual views that provide a context for interpreting the meaning of life changes, illness, and menopause. Failure to address women's spiritual beliefs and concerns can frustrate the shared medical decision-making process because of lack of communication about fundamental issues. Physicians should not exert influence over a woman's spiritual or religious views. However, women should seek a physician that attends to spiritual beliefs in a sensitive manner. In addition, physicians must learn how to appropriately inquire about spiritual issues and to communicate compassion and care for the whole person. They should also learn to initiate referral to a minister, certified chaplain, or other clergy when significant issues are identified.

Should Doctors Address Spiritual Issues
in the Health Care Setting?

One of the most important reasons for physicians to address spirituality is its impact on health-related decisions and behaviors. More than two-thirds of American women state that their religion is the most important influence in their daily lives versus only half of men. Spiritual and religious commitment are more prevalent among women than men. Patients in hospitals express religious and spiritual orientations even more strongly. One survey of patients at two hospitals revealed that three quarters prayed daily or more often. More than 90 percent of all patients and virtually all women surveyed agreed that spiritual health is as important as physical health (King and Bushwick, 1994).

Spiritual health is an important source in coping with stress or illness. Discussing spiritual coping when addressing midlife issues may add an important dimension to the interaction. Whether a woman draws strength from friends, family, or faith, her physician should take the time to inquire and become aware so that he or she can appreciate the patient's views and become more aware of resources available in times of stress.

Medical researchers have documented the importance of coping in seriously ill patients. Furthermore, they have documented that patients who use a religious/spiritual support as part of coping have less depression and better health (Pargament et al., 2004).

How Doctors, Nurses, and Other Health Professionals Can Obtain Information About Spiritual Views from Patients

In the process of asking about medical history, doctors and other health care providers can ask about spiritual values, religious beliefs, spiritual needs and concerns, and whatever gives the patient's life and illness meaning. For significant life changes such as menopause, the questions could include how religious and spiritual views affect health, coping, dealing with spiritual concerns, and whether a minister or other spiritual counselor is available to talk to about these issues.

To explore spiritual contexts, some doctors use the FAITH questionnaire. If your doctor does not, you can ask yourself these questions and perhaps gain important insight into the meaning of your own faith in your life, especially during this significant passage.

In the FAITH questionnaire, the first question asks whether you have a *faith* or religion that is important to you. Your denominational affiliation may influence your particular health beliefs and be of interest to your doctor in deciding on appropriate care.

The next question focuses on how specifically your beliefs *apply* to your health. Are there dietary restrictions or religious customs of which the health care team should be aware? Are there any restrictions about use of blood or blood products? Many religious traditions have customs or rituals about diet, prayer, religious holidays or observances, and other beliefs that may affect medical care.

Determining *involvement* in a faith community is helpful in thinking about your available social and spiritual support. Do you have someone to call for counseling or emotional support? Does your congregation offer classes or support groups for people with illness, divorce, or other life stresses?

Treatment decisions may also depend upon spiritual beliefs. If you are facing a hysterectomy, will your beliefs influence your decisions? Some women must deal with religious questions along with health questions since many religious sects regard childbearing as sacred. If you believe in an afterlife, your perspective may differ from those who do not, and your views may be important in making medical decisions about life and death issues.

Finally, ask yourself about ways your doctor could *help* with your spiritual concerns Some patients may share conflicts or questions with their doctor, request to see the chaplain, ask for prayer, or ask the doctor to pray with them. Many patients may not be comfortable praying with doctors, but you should be able to expect that your doctor will be prepared to respond in a compassionate and knowledgeable fashion about your concerns. Sometimes the most important care your doctor can give you is to listen. You may be surprised to find that your health care provider is interested in your spiritual concerns, and cares about you as a whole person.

Encourage Your Doctor to Ask About Your Spiritual Health

Few physicians have been trained to counsel patients in religious or spiritual matters, but training in such matters is on the rise. Many medical schools have formal or elective courses in spirituality and health (King et al., 2004). Many physicians trained before the 1990s have had no training in the relationship between spirituality and health. Consequently, you may need to bring up the subject of spirituality and health first, or let your doctor know it is okay to address such issues in your care. Recent research has documented that many physicians want to address these issues but lack training (Ellis et al., 1999). Also, they may fear their patients will be alienated by spiritual questions. You may need to make the first move. After all, you are not planning to have a theological debate, just an open conversation to let your doctor know that spiritual issues are important to you. You may be amazed at how your doctor will welcome the interchange.

Chapter 8

Last Word

Take a moment to consider this question: Are your expectations optimistic, neutral, or pessimistic about menopause? Your expectations and feelings may have an impact on how you deal with what lies ahead and how you respond to the challenges of midlife.

How do you feel about your level of control over future events? Your assessment of your own ability to influence future events can have a large effect on how things turn out. Do you feel that a powerful and loving God is watching over you? If so, you are more likely to be positive about the future.

One of our goals with this book has been to allay some of your fears about menopause. We endeavored to also provide you with psychological and spiritual resources to face the challenges of menopause and the midlife. We want you to be able to look at this transition as an opportunity for personal growth and development, not just a hurdle to be overcome. We want to leave you with more optimism and hope for the future. We believe that with some love and encouragement and drawing on your personal and spiritual strength you can be more positive, full of hope, and even an inspiration to your family and others.

Recently, some researchers set out to study women's psychological development during menopause and to examine the relationship between women's appraisal of menopause and symptom reporting (Busch et al., 2003). They examined 130 healthy women annually for five consecutive years using semistructured interviews and a menopausal symptom rating scale. Their results showed that, initially, the majority of the women (57 percent) had neutral beliefs about menopause, 31 percent were pessimistic, and

12 percent were optimistic. Optimistic and neutral expectations were associated with fewer symptoms, whereas the pessimistic appraisal was significantly related to having more symptoms. During the course of menopause an amazing thing happened. The majority of the neutral and pessimistic women reappraised menopause during the study period, and at the last follow-up, 67 percent appraised menopause positively. The majority of women felt that menopause had been a positive experience, despite their more negative initial expectations!

Women who changed their minds toward a more positive view of menopause frequently cited personal growth as a major factor in their new attitude. This points to an astounding conclusion: menopause is a *positive* period for most women.

In conclusion, menopause and the midlife transition period are often psychological and spiritual life events as well as physical and physiological events in women's lives. Although depression, anxiety, feelings of grief, and family change are common, most women who go through menopause are capable of positive growth and a new perspective on life. The physical changes of menopause, although distressing and extremely uncomfortable for many, do not in themselves make women seriously physically ill. Cultural expectations about aging and appearance may have a profound affect on women's self-esteem during this period. Stressors such as personal loss, children leaving home, and new responsibilities of caring for aging parents can be overwhelming. However, learning more about menopause and the midlife transition can provide reassurance and let women know that their feelings, emotions, and strife during this period are normal. We have also seen many women benefit from taking more time during the midlife to revisit the relevance of spiritual and religious beliefs. Spiritual faith and prayer can give women a whole new outlook and even beneficially influence psychological and physical health.

The discussions in the previous chapters have provided new avenues for finding peace, new strategies for resisting stress, and new energy to face the future. Our sincere desire is that you have new hope, a hope that can sustain you through the challenges of midlife and beyond.

Resources

The following resources are listed on the Internet at <www. 4woman.gov/Menopause>.

Government Agencies

Administration on Aging, Office of External Affairs
330 Independence Avenue, SW
Washington, DC 20201
Phone: (202) 401-4541
<www.aoa.dhhs.gov>

Agency for Health Care Policy and Research (AHCPR)
540 Gaither Road
Rockville, MD 20850
Phone: (301) 427-1364
<www.ahrq.gov/ppip/healthywom.htm>

Centers for Disease Control and Prevention
Office of Women's Health
1600 Clifton Road, NE
Atlanta, GA 30333
Phone: (404) 639-2607
<www.cdc.gov>

Food and Drug Administration
Office of Women's Health
Parklawn Building, Room 1561
5600 Fishers Lane
Rockville, MD 20857
Fax: (301) 827-0926

<www.fda.gov/womens/default.htm> and
<www.fda.gov/cder>

National Heart, Lung, and Blood Institute (NHLBI)
9000 Rockville Pike
Bethesda, MD 20892
Phone: (301) 496-4236
Fax: (301) 402-1051

National Institute of Child Health and Human Development
Public Information and Communications
Building 31, Room 2A32
31 Center Drive
Bethesda, MD 20892
Phone: (301) 496-5133
Fax: (301) 496-0500
<www.nih.gov/nichd>

National Institute of Mental Health
Parklawn Building, Room 17-99
5600 Fishers Lane
Rockville, MD 20857
Phone: (301) 443-3673
Fax: (301) 443-2578
<www.nimh.nih.gov>

National Institute on Aging
Public Information Office
Building 31, Room 2C234
Bethesda, MD 20892
Phone: (301) 496-1752
Fax: (301) 496-1072
<www.nih.gov/nia>

National Institutes of Health
U.S. Department of Health and Human Services
<www.nih.gov/PHTindex.htm>

National Women's Health Information Center
U.S. Department of Health and Human Services
Phone: (800) 994-9662
TDD: (888) 220-5446
Fax: (301) 443-2578
<www.4woman.gov/Menopause>

Office of Research on Women's Health
National Institutes of Health
Building 1, Room 201
Bethesda, MD 20892
Phone: (301) 402-1770
Fax: (301) 402-1798
<www4.od.nih.gov/orwh/index.html>

Office on Women's Health
Humphrey Building, Room 730B
200 Independence Avenue, SW
Washington, DC 20201
Phone: (202) 690-7650
Fax: (202) 690-7172
<www.4woman.gov/owh/index.htm>

Substance Abuse and Mental Health Services Administration (SAMHSA)
Parklawn Building, Room 13-99
5600 Fishers Lane
Rockville, MD 20857
Phone: (301) 443-5184
Fax: (301) 443-8964

Private Organizations

American College of Obstetricians and Gynecologists (ACOG)
409 12th Street, SW
Washington, DC 20024-2188
Phone: (202) 638-5577
<www.acog.org>

American Menopause Foundation, Inc
The Empire State Building
350 5th Avenue, Suite 822
New York, NY 10118
Phone: (212) 714-2398
<www.americanmenopause.org>

Association of Women's Health, Obstetric and Neonatal Nurses
2000 L Street, NW, Suite 740
Washington, DC 20036
Phone: (202) 261-2400
<www.awhonn.org>

Black Women's Health Imperative
600 Pennsylvania Avenue, SE, Suite 310
Washington, DC 20003
Phone: (202) 548-4000
<www.blackwomenshealth.org/site/PageServer>

Boston Women's Health Book Collective
240A Elm Street
Somerville, MA 02144
Phone: (617) 625-0271
<www.ourbodiesourselves.org>

Hormone Foundation
8401 Connecticut Avenue, Suite 900

Chevy Chase, MD 20815-5817
Phone: (800) 467-6663
<www.hormone.org>

The Jean Mayer USDA Human Nutrition Research Center on Aging
Tufts University
711 Washington Street
Boston, MA 02111
Phone: (617) 556-3000
Fax: (617) 556-3344
<www.hnrc.tufts.edu>

Melpomene Institute
1010 University Avenue
St. Paul, MN 55104
Phone: (612) 642-1951
<www.melpomene.org>

National Center on Women and Aging
Brandeis University
Waltham, MA 02254-9110
Phone: (800) 929-1995
Fax: (781) 736 3866
<www.heller.brandeis.edu/national/>

National Osteoporosis Foundation (NOF)
1232 22nd Street, NW, Suite 602
Washington, DC 20037
Phone: (202) 223-2226
<www.nof.org>

National Women's Health Network
514 10th Street, NW, Suite 400
Washington, DC 20004
Phone: (202) 628-7814

North American Menopause Society (NAMS)
PO Box 94527
Cleveland, OH 44101
Phone: (440) 442-7550
<www.menopause.org>

Older Women's League
1750 New York Avenue, NW, Suite 350
Washington, DC 20006
Phone: (202) 783-6686
<www.owl-national.org>

Osteoporosis and Related Bone Diseases National Resource Center
1232 22nd Street, NW
Washington, DC 20037
Phone: (800) 624-BONE
<www.osteo.org>

Planned Parenthood Federation of America
434 West 33rd Street
New York, NY 10001
Phone: (212) 541-7800

Newsletters, Magazines, and Reports

Hot Flash: A Newsletter for Midlife and Older Women
The National Action Forum for Midlife and Older Women
Box 816
Stony Brook, NY 11790-0609

Menopause Flashes
The North American Menopause Society

Menopause News
Judith Askew, Editor
2074 Union Street, Suite 10
San Francisco, CA 94123

Osteoporosis Report
National Osteoporosis Foundation
2100 M Street, NW, Suite 602
Washington, DC 20037
Phone: (202) 223-2226

Selected Bibliography

Introduction

Carver CS, Pozo C, and Harris SD (1993). How coping mediates the effect of optimism on distress: A study of women with early stage breast cancer. *Journal of Personality and Social Psychology* 65: 375-390.

Johnson SC and Spilka B (1991). Coping with breast cancer: The roles of clergy and faith. *Journal of Religion and Health* 30: 21-33.

King DE (2000). *Faith, Spirituality, and Medicine: Toward the Making of a Healing Practitioner*. Binghamton, NY: The Haworth Press.

Koenig HG, McCullough M, and Larson DB (2001). *Handbook of Religion and Health*. New York: Oxford University Press.

Northrup C (1997). Menopause. *Primary Care* 24(4): 921-948.

Chapter 1. The Transition to Menopause: The Journey Begins

Bosworth HB, Bastian LA, Rimer BK, and Siegler IC (2003). Coping styles and personality domains related to menopausal stress. *Women's Health Issues* 13: 32-38.

Buchanan MC, Villagran MM, and Ragan SL (2002). Women, menopause, and (Ms.)Information: Communication about the climacteric. *Health Communication* 14(1): 99-119.

Ferguson SJ and Parry C (1998). Rewriting menopause: Challenging the medical paradigm to reflect menopausal women's experiences. *Frontiers* 19(1): 20-41.

Leidy LE, Canali C, and Callahan WE (2000). The medicalization of menopause: Implications for recruitment of study participants. *Menopause* 7(3): 193-199.

Reynolds F (2002). Exploring self-image during hot flushes using a semantic differential scale: Associations between poor self-image, depression, flush frequency, and flush distress. *Maturitas* 42(3): 201-207.

Rice F and Furth J (1994). Menopause and the working boomer. *Fortune* 130(10): 203 (6 pages).

Sheehy G (1998). *The Silent Passage*. New York: Simon & Schuster.

Woods NF (1998). Menopause: Models, medicine, and mid-life. *Frontiers* 19(1): 5-19.

Chapter 2. Closing and Opening Doors: Dealing with a Journey of Personal Loss

Carter E and McGoldrick M (1989). *Changing Family Life Cycle: A Framework for Family Therapy*, Second edition. Boston: Allyn & Bacon.

Doress-Worters PB and Laskin SD (1987). *Ourselves, Growing Older: Women Aging with Knowledge and Power*. New York: Simon & Schuster.

Morrow LA (1975). *Gift from the Sea*. New York: Pantheon Books.

Utian WH and Boggs PP (1999). The North American Menopause Society 1998 Menopause Survey: Part I. Postmenopausal women's perceptions about menopause and mid-life. *Menopause* 6: 122-128.

Van Eyk McCain M (1991). *Transformation Through Menopause*. New York: Bergin & Garvey.

Wall K and Ferguson G (1998). *Rites of Passage: Celebrating Life's Changes*. Hillsboro, OR: Beyond Words Publishing.

Warren R (2002). *The Purpose-Driven Life: What on Earth am I Here For?* Grand Rapids, MI: Zondervan.

Chapter 3. Mood and the Mind in Menopause

Bhatia S (1999). Depression in women: Diagnostic and treatment considerations. *American Family Physician* 60(1): 225-240.

Brown CS (2001). Depression and anxiety disorders. *Obstetrics and Gynecology Clinics of North America* 28(2): 241-268.

Cobb, JO (1998). Reasssuring the woman facing menopause: Strategies and resources. *Patient Education and Counseling* 33: 281-288.

Dosey MF and Dosey MA (1980). The climacteric woman. *Patient Counseling and Health Education* 2(1): 14-21.

Fitzpatrick LA and Santen RJ (2002). Hot flashes: The old and the new. What is really true? *Mayo Clinic Proceedings* 77(11): 1-4.

Huston JE and Lanka LD (1997). *Perimenopause: Changes in Women's Health After 35*. Oakland, CA: New Harbinger Publications, Inc.

Koenig HG, George LK, and Peterson BL (1998). Religiosity and remission from depression in medically ill older patients. *American Journal of Psychiatry* 155: 536-542.

Nijs P (1998). Counseling of the climacteric woman: Diagnostic difficulties and therapeutic possibilities. *European Journal of Obstetrics and Gynecology* 81: 273-276.

Northrup C (1997). Menopause. *Primary Care* 24(4): 921-948.

Propst LR, Ostrom R, Watkins P, Dean T, and Mashburn D (1992). Comparative efficacy of religious and non-religious cognitive-behavioral therapy for the treatment of clinical depression in religious individuals. *Journal of Consulting and Clinical Psychology* 60: 94-103.

Woods NF and Mitchell ES (1999). Anticipating menopause: Observations from the Seattle Midlife Women's Health Study. *Menopause* 6(2): 167-173.

Chapter 4. Counseling and Group Support

Bhatia S (1999). Depression in women: Diagnostic and treatment considerations. *American Family Physician* 60(1): 225-240.

Brown CS (2001). Depression and anxiety disorders. *Obstetrics and Gynecology Clinics of North America* 28(2): 241-268.

Cobb JO (1998). Reassuring the woman facing menopause: Strategies and resources. *Patient Education and Counseling* 33: 281-288.

Dosey MF and Dosey MA (1980). The climacteric woman. *Patient Counseling and Health Education* 2(1): 14-21.

Nijs P (1998). Counseling of the climacteric woman: Diagnostic difficulties and therapeutic possibilities. *European Journal of Obstetrics and Gynecology* 81: 273-276.

Reddy H (1971). "I Am Woman." Irving Music, Inc., OBO Itself and Buggerlugs Music Company.

Chapter 5. Exercise: Moving Along the Menopause Journey

Centers for Disease Control and Prevention, National Center for Chronic Disease Prevention and Health Promotion (2003). Nutrition and Physical Activity. Available at: <www.cdc.gov/nccdphp/dnpa/physical/index.htm>.

Dunn AL, Andersen RE, and Jakicic JM (1998). Lifestyle physical activity interventions: History, short- and long-term effects, and recommendations. *American Journal of Preventive Medicine* 15(4): 398-412.

Dunn AL, Marcus BH, Kampert JB, Garcia ME, Kohl HW, and Blair SN (1999). Comparison of lifestyle and structured interventions to increase physical activity and cardiorespiratory fitness: A randomized trial. *Journal of the American Medical Association* 281(4): 327-334.

Hammermeister JJ, Page RM, and Dolny D (2000). Psychosocial, behavioral, and biometric characteristics of stages of exercise adoption. *Psychological Reports* 87(1): 205-217.

Laforge RG, Rossi JS, Prochaska JO, Velicer WF, Levesque DA, and McHorney CA (1999). Stage of regular exercise and health-related quality of life. *Preventive Medicine* 28(4): 349-360.

Litt MD, Kleppinger A, and Judge JO (2002). Initiation and maintenance of exercise behavior in older women: Predictors from the social learning model. *Journal of Behavioral Medicine* 25(1): 83-97.

Lovejoy JC (1998). The influence of sex hormones on obesity across the female life span. *Journal of Women's Health* 7(10): 1247-1256.

Stutts WC (2002). Physical activity determinates in adults: Perceived benefits, barriers, and self efficacy. *American Association of Occupational Health Nurses Journal* 50(11): 499-507.

Chapter 6. Menopause and the Workplace

Benson H and Klipper MZ (1975). *The Relaxation Response.* New York: William Morrow and Company.

Menopause Online (2003). "Focusing" and Menopause. Available at: <www.menopause-online.com/focusing.htm>.

Ramsland KM (2000). *Bliss: Writing to Find Your True Self.* Cincinnati, OH: Walking Stick Press.

Rice F and Furth J (1994). Menopause and the working boomer. *Fortune* 130(10): 203.

Senior World Online (2003). Managing Menopause in the Corporate Workplace. Available at: <www.seniorworld.com/articles/a19990816182741.html>.

Sheehy G (1998). *The Silent Passage.* New York: Simon & Schuster.

Witkowski JM (2003). Relieving Stress 101—Simple Yoga in the Workplace. University Health Systems, Berkeley, CA. Retrieved September 30, 2003, from <www.uhs.berkeley.edu/HealthInfo/EdHandouts/menopause.htm>.

Woods NF (1998). Menopause: Models, medicine, and midlife. *Frontiers* 19(1): 5-19.

Chapter 7. Spiritual Issues Facing Women at Midlife

Alcorn R (2003). *The Grace and Truth Paradox.* Sisters, OR: Mulnomah Publishers.

Anandarajah G and Hight E (2000). Spirituality and medical practice: Using the HOPE questions as a practical tool for spiritual assessment. *American Family Physician* 63: 81-88.

Carver CS, Pozo C, and Harris SD (1993). How coping mediates the effect of optimism on distress: A study of women with early stage breast cancer. *Journal of Personality and Social Psychology* 65: 375-390.

Dedert EA, Studts JL, Weissbecker I, Salmon PG, Banis PL, and Sephton SE (2004). Religiosity may help preserve the cortisol rhythm in women with stress-related illness. *International Journal of Psychiatry in Medicine* 34(1): 61-77.

Ellis MR, Vinson DC, and Ewigman B (1999). Addressing spiritual concerns of patients: Family physicians' attitudes and practices. *Journal of Family Practice* 48(2): 105-109.

Harmon RL and Myers MA (1999). Prayer and meditation as medical therapies. *Physical Medicine and Rehabilitation Clinics of North America* 10(3): 651-662.

Hummer RA, Rogers RG, Nam CB, and Ellison CG (1999). Religious involvement and U.S. adult mortality. *Demography* 36(2): 273-285.

Ironson G, Solomon GF, Balbin EG, O'Cleirigh C, George A, Kumar M, Larson D, and Woods TE (2002). The Ironson-Woods Spirituality/Religiousness Index is associated with long survival, health behaviors, less distress, and low cortisol in people with HIV/AIDS. *Annals of Behavioral Medicine* 24(1): 34-48.

Johnson SC and Spilka B (1991). Coping with breast cancer: The roles of clergy and faith. *Journal of Religion and Health* 30: 21-33.

Jones J (1994). Embodied meaning: Menopause and the change of life. *Social Work in Health Care* 19: 43-65.

King DE (2000). *Faith, Spirituality, and Medicine: Toward the Making of a Healing Practitioner*. Binghamton, NY: The Haworth Press.

King DE (2002). Spirituality and medicine. In MB Mengel, WL Holleman, and S Fields (Eds.), *Fundamentals of Clinical Practice: A Textbook on the Patient, Doctor, and Society* (pp. 651-670). New York: Kluwer.

King DE, Blue A, Mallin R, and Thiedke C (2004). Implementation and assessment of a spiritual history taking curriculum in the first year of medical school. *Teaching and Learning in Medicine* 16(1): 64-68.

King DE and Bushwick B (1994). Beliefs and attitudes of hospital inpatients about faith healing and prayer. *Journal of Family Practice* 39(4): 349-352.

King DE, Mainous AG 3rd, and Pearson WS (2002). C-reactive protein, diabetes, and attendance at religious services. *Diabetes Care* 25(7): 1172-1176.

King DE, Mainous AG 3rd, Steyer TE, and Pearson W (2001). The relationship between attendance at religious services and cardiovascular inflammatory markers. *International Journal of Psychiatry in Medicine* 31(4): 415-425.

Koenig HG, Cohen HJ, Blazer DG, Kudler HS, Krishnan KR, and Sibert TE (1995). Religious coping and depression among elderly, hospitalized, medically ill men. *Psychosomatics* 36(4): 369-375.

Koenig HG, George LK, and Peterson BL (1998). Religiosity and remission from depression in medically ill older patients. *American Journal of Psychiatry* 155: 536-542.

Koenig HG, McCullough M, and Larson DB (2001). *Handbook of Religion and Health*. New York: Oxford University Press.

Larimore W (2003). *10 Essentials of Highly Healthy People*. Grand Rapids, MI: Zondervan.

Levin J (2002). Is depressed affect a function of one's relationship with God? Findings from a study of primary care patients. *International Journal of Psychiatry in Medicine* 32(4): 379-393.

MacNutt F (1974, 1999). *Healing*. Notre Dame, IN: Ave Maria Press.

Matthews DA, McCullough ME, Larson DB, Koenig HG, Swyers JP, and Milano MG (1998). Religious commitment and health status: A review of the research and implications for family medicine. *Archives of Family Medicine* 7(2): 118-124.

McCullough ME, Fincham FD, and Tsang J (2003). Forgiveness, forbearance, and time: The temporal unfolding of transgression-related interpersonal motivations. *The Journal of Personality and Social Psychology* 84(3): 540-557.

Musick MA, House JS, and Williams DR (2004). Attendance at religious services and mortality in a national sample. *Journal of Health and Social Behavior* 45(2): 198-213.

Northrup C (2001). *The Wisdom of Menopause*. New York: Bantam Books.

Oman D and Reed D (1998). Religion and mortality among the community-dwelling elderly. *American Journal of Public Health* 88(10): 1469-1475.

Pargament KI, Koenig HG, Tarakeshwar N, and Hahn J (2004). Religious coping methods as predictors of psychological, physical, and spiritual outcomes among medically ill elderly patients: A two-year longitudinal study. *Journal of Health Psychology* 9(6): 713-730.

Pennebaker JW and Seagal JD (1999). Forming a story: The health benefits of narrative. *Journal of Clinical Psychology* 55(10): 1243-1254.

Chapter 8. Last Word

Busch H, Barth-Olofsson AS, Rosenhagen S, and Collins A (2003). Menopausal transition and psychological development. *Menopause* 10: 179-187.

Index

Page numbers followed by the letter "b" indicate boxed text; those followed by the letter "t" indicate tables.